Primal Scream

A cry in the night
not like the worried whistling of a hare
or the sorrowful lament of a deer
A cry as old as time itself
the wild growling of a mother bear in her cave
like loud thunder in the mountains
unrestrained like the stormy sea
Lightning as if the sky touched the earth
then silence
and in that silence
the quiet cry of a newborn

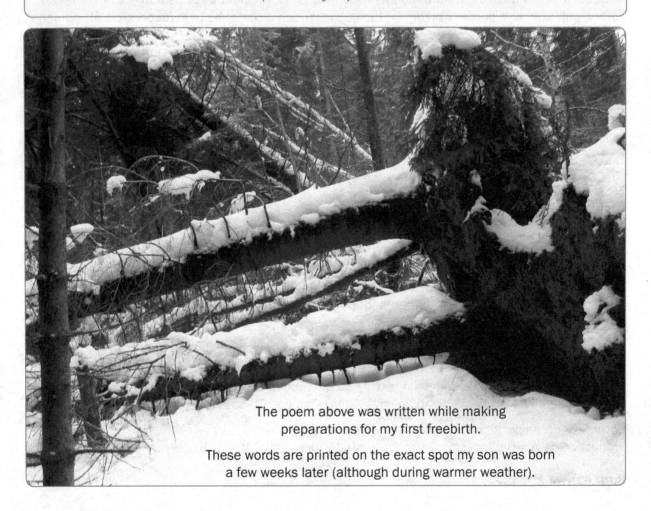

The poem above was written while making
preparations for my first freebirth.

These words are printed on the exact spot my son was born
a few weeks later (although during warmer weather).

Bibliografische Information der Deutschen Nationalbibliothek

Die Deutsche Nationalbibliothek verzeichnet diese Publikation in der Deutschen Nationalbibliografie; detaillierte bibliografische Daten sind im Internet über http://dnb.d-nb.de abrufbar.

Disclaimer of liability

Any queries regarding healthcare during pregnancy and birth should be answered by a healthcare professional. Advice and suggestions in this book are not intended to replace medical advice. If in doubt, please consult your midwife, gynaecologist, doctor or pharmacist. Parts of this book are based on numerous reports of personal experience and to maintain authenticity we could not modify the content in any way. Author, editors, guest authors or the publisher cannot be held responsible for any damages or disadvantages resulting from the contents of this book. All information is subject to change. The author, publisher and people working for the publisher can also not be held responsible for personal, material and financial damage.

Should there be errors in this book, despite our careful proofreading, please let the publisher know in writing.

Trademark protection

This book contains brand names and trade names. Usual conditions apply even if they are not marked as such.

First German edition	July 2014, „Alleingeburt – Schwangerschaft und Geburt in Eigenregie"
First English edition	April 2015, translated by Deborah Neiger (Midwife)

© 2014–2015	edition riedenburg
Address	edition riedenburg, Anton-Hochmuth-Strasse 8, 5020 Salzburg, Austria
E-Mail	verlag@editionriedenburg.at
Internet	editionriedenburg.at
Editors	Dr. Heike Wolter, Regensburg; Anna Rockel-Loenhoff, Unna (German edition) Elizabeth Hormann IBCLC (English edition)
Design	Fotolia.com: Coverphoto © EpicStockMedia; Illustr. on page 38 © ngaga35; Wavegraphics at the start of each chapter © lukeruk
	Body sketches: © Sarah Schmid
	Photos in main text: © Sarah Schmid except for the placenta photos (top and bottom right) on page 104 © Caroline Oblasser

Coverdesign, composition and layout: edition riedenburg
Production (D, A, CH): Books on Demand GmbH, Norderstedt • Also available in the UK / USA

ISBN 978-3-902943-86-6

Sarah Schmid

Freebirth

Self-Directed Pregnancy and Birth

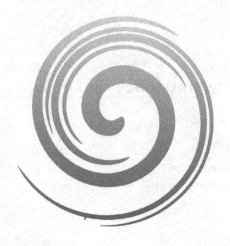

Translated from German
by Deborah Neiger (Midwife)

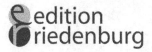
edition
riedenburg

Contents

Freebirth – Mothers tell their stories   **139**

Appendix   **231**

Introduction

In the beginning ...

Our life on this earth starts with birth and ends with death. We are all born and we all die at some point. There is nothing which touches us more in our being than birth and death, the beginning and end of our life.

To take away some of the threat of mortality, humankind has introduced rituals, traditions and taboos. Standard procedures that reassure us when there is nothing else to reassure. This book is about birthing and about the time in which a woman is 'with child'. About the time in which we would like to drift in the sea of life in the expectation of new horizons, if it weren't for all the health warnings and advice from well meaning people on the shore.

When people hear that a woman has birthed her baby – without hospital, without midwives or any other help, possibly even intentionally – they are usually incredulous.

How daring! Isn't it extremely dangerous, irresponsible even? How does the woman know what to do? What does she do with the umbilical cord?

The reaction is much less dramatic, trite even, when telling the exact same story about a cat. Even though she has done exactly the same: without hospital, without midwife, without help. All by herself.

And generally she won't have just birthed one baby, but four or five. In a dusty, or at least non sterile, corner in the house. She opened the amniotic sacs of her babies one by one and ate them, severed the umbilical cords and licked every newborn clean.

After this loving welcome, one kitten after the other crawled along mama's cosy fur and found a teat, on which it will spend many snuggly hours from now on.

Didn't this mother cat do well? She never had any notes or an estimated date of birth. No one listened to her babies' heartbeats or monitored her contractions. No one checked her dilatation. No one told her when to start pushing.

No one protected her perineum or prepared a coffee compress. She also didn't prepare for birth by massaging her own perineum in the weeks preceding birth. And she also didn't attend a course on how to look after a bunch of newborn kittens.

Despite all this, she knew exactly what to do, instinctively. And what did she need to be able to do this? Nothing. Except for a quiet, dry place.

It is not only cats who birth like this. Birds, rabbits, mice, foxes, deer, monkeys and elephants seek out a safe place for the birth of their babies: a nest in a tree, a cave, a crack in a rockface, a grassy den or, alternatively, they are surrounded by members of their pack or herd. This is where they birth their offspring protected from predators and interruptions, entirely unspectacularly, without technical surveillance or medical help, under their own steam. Freebirth is a tried and tested phenomenon in the animal kingdom.

Only we humans somehow fall out of this norm, especially the modern human. Is that because evolution made us walk upright and gave us bigger heads for our growing intelligence and therefore made birth more difficult?

But how do we explain all the reports from different indigenous people (during a time when they were hardly touched by Western civilisation) about quick, effortless births that astonished so many Western observers? Births alone in a remote hut, alone during the night, during work in the fields, births in the presence of a trusted wise woman ... easy births certainly seemed the norm rather than the exception.

Why this was possible then and not now is not the subject of research trials, however. No one believes that a quick, easy, joyful birth is possible anyway.

We would much rather advocate quick pain relief in the form of an epidural to render a woman's abdomen and pelvis without sensation.

The impression is that easy births are rare. Positive births are all about luck, and maybe it's not really all that important anyway. 'The main thing is that the baby is healthy.' is a saying heard often.

Does it not matter anymore how women experience birth in modern society? In the name of safety and responsibility for our children, women are often deprived of a positive and empowering birth experience. Why take risks and trust mother nature when expensive technology, experienced doctors and close monitoring can do a better job?

My journey to freebirth

My first foray into modern obstetrics happened before my first pregnancy. During my time in medical school I had various shorter placements in hospitals as well as a whole year at a later point in my studies.

I knew I wanted to have children and used the opportunity to take up a placement in the obstetrics and gynaecology department of my local hospital. I didn't have any preconceived ideas about birth, was curious and excited about every birth I was allowed to attend. Once I even saw twins born. And once, but only once did I witness a birth in an upright position, rather than with the woman on her back, as usual. I observed the organisation of the nursery and assisted with caesarean sections. I had to suction the amniotic fluid as soon as the amniotic sac was opened.

The doctors were all relatively nice. The midwives were all very different. I still remember one very young midwife who attended the upright kneeling birth mentioned above with me. Her cheeks always turned bright red as birth approached and she never had to check the mother's cervix to know it was fully dilated. This gut feeling impressed me amidst all the technology and monitoring.

My next experience of obstetrics was during my year long placement. I was married by then, pregnant with my first baby and was therefore hardly allowed to do anything clinical such as take bloods. Watching was allowed though and watch I did.

This time my placement was in the biggest hospital in town. I spent two month in the very labour ward I was born in myself. The midwives were the type famous in the former East Germany and tone in general was regimental.

The women were shouted at and insulted if they didn't follow the midwives' instructions. A generous episiotomy was routine and seemed very painful although the women were usually reassured that it wouldn't be. The student midwives tried to trump each other with the the numbers of episiotomies they had performed.

There were many situations I found horrifying and the decision to have a homebirth was an easy one. The risk of having to birth in this hospital was not one I was willing to take. My husband was in agreement as the hospital was only 5 minutes away from our house at the edge of the woods and was easily accessible in the case of an emergency.

Through recommendation I found and older, experienced midwife. I had a good feeling about her and felt like nothing could go wrong. The year long placement I was doing at the time was very stressful. 4 months of it took place in Accident and Emergency. It was exciting and educational but I got very constipated.

I found a very reliable remedy for this, which brought relief in 15 minutes flat: the forest. As soon as I went for a walk there, I felt like everything started to move again, as it were. As I wandered amongst the trees and felt relief take over, I thought again and again: I have to birth my baby right here. I'm just going to escape, without anyone knowing where I am and come back with a baby. No trouble, no stress, no expectations, demands or clocks. That would be amazing. If I can get rid of constipation so easily here, it must be the ideal place to push out a baby.

While I pondered this, I came to the conclusion that it just would not be practical. Too many people out running and walking their dogs and at the end of the day there really was nowhere secluded enough. Despite that, the thought stayed with me.

So our first child was born in our rented flat and not in the forest. I thought I had done everything I could to achieve a positive birth and felt positive. As my estimated date of birth passed I refused to go for monitoring with a CTG (a machine that records the fetal heart as well as uterine activity) every other day.

My midwife thought I might be the type of woman who might well birth alone and call her out too late. And she was right. Secretly I had considered that as an option. But because we wanted to be nice, we called her in the morning to say that contractions had started, just to give her the heads up. Then, two things happened we wouldn't have been able to predict: our midwife was at another birth and the back up midwife from the birth center turned up at our flat despite us telling her we didn't need anyone yet.

So there she was, the back up midwife. I didn't click with her and just wanted her to go away as quickly as possible. She was on the way out again, leaving us the phone number we could reach her under, when ... suddenly my contractions became a lot stronger. She stayed. Unfortunately I didn't have the courage and nerve to throw her out and thought: grit your teeth and get it over with.

But this didn't quite turn out as I'd hoped. Soon I was fully dilated and a second midwife was called in anticipation of the birth as is common during homebirths. Then I didn't progress for hours. Only contractions and pain. PAIN! And then, after careful palpation the realisation: the head was engaged but had not rotated into the right position.

Now the sword of Damocles 'Caesarean in hospital' hung over me. I had surrendered the responsibility for my birth to the midwives and they also didn't know what to do in this situation. Realising that they were clueless, it became clear I needed to take back my power and do whatever could save me from the operating table. If my body knew how to get the baby out, I needed to listen to it, not to the midwives with their seemingly ineffective advice to lie down and change position from the right to the left and back to the right frequently.

So I listened intently to my body and instinctually started moving my hips from side to side while standing and encouraging my daughter to move into a better position. Luckily, this is when MY midwife arrived. She massaged my swollen anterior lip of cervix (very painful but effective). The baby's head had finally turned and soon I was holding my baby in my arms. Completely exhausted but very very happy.

After the initial oxytocin haze I started to analyse the birth. What went wrong? How could I have avoided all those hours of pain? Why was it that everything became so much more difficult as soon as the midwife arrived?

I read voraciously on the internet, informed myself about freebirths and it didn't take long until I had an epiphany. I was obviously not the only one who was affected so profoundly by the presence of certain people that an undisturbed birth became impossible.

Apparently, inviting strangers to one's birth can be a risk in itself.

At the same time I asked myself: If I ever had another baby, how could I make that birth a positive one? How could I be sure that the person attending me wouldn't inhibit me, mistrust my body or take away the emotional strength I needed to birth my baby?

I slowly came to the determination that my next birth would only be attended by people who did not fear birth. Would I find someone like that?

Shortly after the birth of our daughter, we moved to Sweden. Directly behind our house a deserted forest sprawled and I only had to go out the back door to relieve my constipation.

One day, on a stroll through the forest, I found it: the place our son was to be born. The ground was covered in soft moss and it was surrounded with fallen spruce trees mimicking walls. Next to it was a babbling brook. The forest was wild here, no hikers, mushroom collectors or runners ever to be seen. I was thrilled! From then on I made my way to this place frequently and imagined what birthing there would be like ...

Once my husband had come round to the idea of birth in the wild I led him to my place.

My second pregnancy was very different to my first. I was just pregnant.

Antenatal care in my first pregnancy, specifically the frequent scans, had unsettled and irritated me. Now I was completely free and organised care for myself. Unbelievably freeing. I did, however, also have periods of doubt on this new path. Where would this decision to do my own maternity care lead me?

I was well and I could feel my baby move inside me, so I kept following my path. At first I considered going to the traditional appointments from a certain point in my pregnancy but as the point approached, I bristled. I felt like my bubble was going to burst if a stranger started measuring and judging our progress.

At some point I dropped the plan to access traditional care and was pleased to avoid the stress.

I had given up in my search for the perfect homebirth midwife ages ago. First of all there are hardly any homebirth midwives in Sweden and she would have had to travel far to reach me and secondly I would have had to pay EU2000 for her to attend the birth with no guarantee that she would actually be able to get to me on time. Thirdly, I would have had to convince the midwife of my forest birth plans.

So I did it without a midwife. And because I liked it so much I did the same for my third, fourth and fifth babies.

My medical degree played only a small role in my decision to walk this path alone. My studies did help me to see obstetrics with all its limitations and not to have false expectations.

As it stands we still haven't uncovered all the secrets of life. We still can't explain how the immune system works exactly or have the knowledge to eradicate common diseases like cancer or allergies.

When it comes to birth, medicine has a lot to learn still. We use an arsenal of monitoring tools and medical interventions to compensate for what we don't understand about true physiological birth, which in turn hinders or even halts the process of birth. And all this not because birth is so complicated, but because it seems so unpredictable that even experienced birth professionals fear it all their lives – fear that has to be eased with many interventions.

Luckily I know someone who knows exactly how birth works: my body. And it has proven this to me five times so far.

This is why I will always listen to my body to achieve a positive and safe birth. I don't want someone to make decisions for me when I can make better ones for myself.

Read on the next few pages how I experienced the freebirths of my second, third, fourth and fifth babies:

My first freebirth (second baby)

A good year after our eldest was born I was pregnant again. We had since moved to Sweden and I was yearning for a birth without anyone in attendance. My husband was less convinced. He had his doubts until the end.

My EDB was the 1st of July. After a false start just before that date contractions started a week later. I was lying in bed on the 8th of July at 11pm and felt a 'pop'.

I stuffed a towel between my legs, finished writing in my diary and thought: how interesting that it is starting like this! I told my husband, and because I could feel more and more amniotic fluid draining, I finally got into the shower where even more waters gushed out.

We were giggling like overexcited teenagers, but because nothing else was happening, we decided to go to bed as usual and try to get some sleep.

I couldn't sleep though. The baby was awake and moving around and contractions came every 5 minutes. I didn't have to consciously breathe through them yet but lying down was uncomfortable. I roamed the house.

Everyone was asleep and I felt anxious not to disturb anyone. Around midnight I went into the garden. It was quiet, I could smell the flowers and both our cats kept me company.

I vocalised through the more and more intense contractions, walked around, visited our rabbits and sat at the edge of the patio. As contractions got stronger and stronger I felt the need to go to my special birth place.

I had a basket that contained everything I felt I might need for the birth and with that I walked the 5 minutes along the forest path until I reached my spot. With its fallen trees, round stones and soft moss it seemed just as perfect for birth as it had months before.

I spread out the picnic blanket, listened to the silence around me and thought how very surreal this moment felt.

The contractions of transition came soon, and the initial chill soon disappeared. I couldn't stay still during contractions. After a tough transition and a few pushes, the head was born. The baby did an almighty kick inside me, I felt the shoulders turn and – whoosh – he was out.

I could just about see that it was 3.19am on this early Swedish summer morning.

A boy! I lifted him up, felt his heart beating and rubbed him dry. He didn't cry, but looked around curiously. I wrapped him in a towel, took a photo and called my husband on my mobile. He arrived shortly after and already knew we had a son by looking at his face.

We slowly walked back to the house. After a few steps I birthed the placenta on the forest floor.

At home I had a shower, we snuggled into bed and slept the rest of the night until morning.

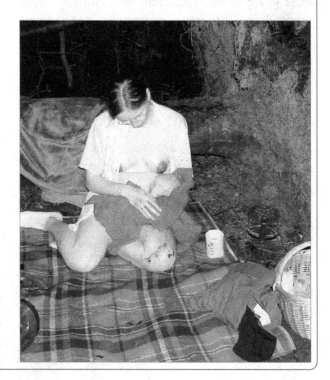

My second freebirth (third baby)

My third pregnancy, a little over a year later, was uncomplicated and again, I didn't have any official antenatal care. My EDB was the 31st of May.

I assumed I would go over my dates again which is why I assumed the very noticable contractions on the 30th and 31st were of no significance. The false alarm from my previous pregnancy was still fresh in my mind. The contractions on the 31st were much stronger than the ones on the day before though.

As I was putting the kids to bed at 9pm I had to breathe through the contractions. My husband took over after 15 minutes. I went to answer some emails and told everyone on the homebirth forum of my harmless but regular contractions. Shortly after 10pm my husband came downstairs and suggested we shower and go to bed as normal and see what happened in the meantime.

In the bathroom I was cold and sweaty at the same time, my legs were shaky. My husband was concerned and asked if this was normal. I reassured him: Yes, this is normal in transition.

My rational brain had realised: Transition. But I hadn't really taken it in. It was far too early. The contractions felt far too weak. Anyway, we still wanted to take belly pictures and I had a shopping trip planned for the next day.

We decided to take some belly pics. We managed three during which I was complaining that a birth here and now was really not convenient. During the last picture I needed to push. I realised I needed a poo and ran towards the toilet. Next urge to push at the bathroom door and my waters went.

Now I realised. But I wanted to birth in our tipi in the garden! We put it up especially. So I grabbed the bag with birthy paraphernalia I had put together throughout the day and ran.

A few meters into the garden I needed to push again. A few steps further the next contraction and I could feel the head already. I was 15m away from our tipi but I could not move.

Finally my husband appeared. He brought coal and lighters to make the tipi cosy and luckily he also brought the video camera. Soon the head was born and with the next contraction, the whole little guy. I squatted down and let him slip into the grass. It was 10.56pm.

I picked him up and he looked at me with big eyes. We covered him with a towel as he started to complain about the cold. Then we sat in the grass and looked on in wonder.

It had been so quick.

Finally we went back to the house. The placenta had come out on the grass. Then I showered and all three of us snuggled into bed.

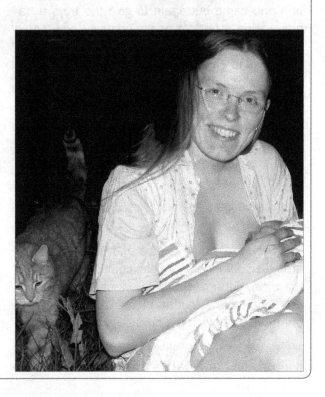

My third freebirth (fourth baby)

My fourth pregnancy, again a year later, went by without problems and without antenatal care.

Five days after my EDB I had a few definite contractions throughout the afternoon, just as I did a few days before. They got stronger in the night so I had to breathe through them but stayed 15 to 30 minutes apart, too far apart for imminent birth.

I forced myself to stay in bed and sleep in between contractions. At about 2am I couldn't bear to lie down anymore. I started to prepare the living room – it was too cold for an outside birth at the beginning of April. But while I sorted and tidied the contractions disappeared. So I went back to bed, where they came back in the same intensity as before.

Same the next morning. Occasional strong contractions. Soon it became harder and harder to fulfil the children's demands and breathe through contractions at the same time.

Again and again I escaped into the bathroom, locked myself in to breathe through a contraction and came out again to give the boys a banana, wipe a bottom or do whatever else small things need doing every minute with small children around. Now the contractions were closer together and required some vocalisation. The boys started to bother me.

Annoyingly, grandma was fairly far away that day and the back up, our neighbour, could not be reached. So my husband suggested he take the children away so I could birth in peace.

Such a suggestion from my husband! I was amazed.

But who would take photos and film? And I had promised our eldest that she could be present for the birth, but now she irritated me so much with her defiant behaviour that I just wanted to get rid of her together with the boys.

My husband eventually reached another neighbour. Around 11.30am she took the boys over.

The eldest was allowed to stay after promising to behave.

Finally there was peace and quiet in the house. I paced the living room. My husband returned quickly and settled down with our eldest and a book. Soon I was drawn into the playroom next door. I didn't want to be watched during the powerful contractions of transition. I tried singing which had always helped a lot but this time it brought no relief.

Then the first contraction that felt a bit pushy at the end. Finally!

'You can start filming now.' I let my husband know. Pushing felt best with me leaning onto something while standing up. It was hard, powerful and not entirely pain free.

Then I felt the head and in the next moment our baby slipped into my hands. A girl! We all marvelled at her, not least her proud big sister.

Then grandma came. She got the boys from the neighbour's house and they got to admire their little sister within an hour of her birth.

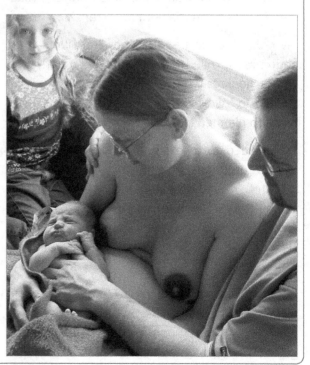

My fourth freebirth (fifth baby)

My fifth pregnancy, a little over 2 years later, was entirely unremarkable, just like the others and I was able to enjoy it – after the tendency towards sinus infections in the first few weeks, already familiar to me – until the very last day of being pregnant.

I didn't even encounter problems with my weak pelvic floor or painful joints – probably thanks to my standing work desk and therefore the avoidance of non ergonomic sitting.

We had been living in Alsace for a year, which means closer to areas with good midwifery care provision. However, in reality, the state of homebirth midwifery is nearly as abysmal here as it was in Sweden, and I didn't really need a midwife anyway.

Because my belly was rather big very early in this pregnancy I let a midwife have a feel around the middle of pregnancy to make sure I knew how many little ones were growing in there. It turned out to be only the one baby. What I could feel turned out to be uterine muscle which was much more developed in this fifth pregnancy than it was before.

Apart from this appointment with the midwife, I was happy doing my own antenatal care. I calculated this baby to be due in January – a winter baby.

One day past my due date I lay awake at night with regular contractions coming every seven minutes. I nearly needed to breathe through them but when morning came everything calmed down again.

My uterus only became noticeably active 6 days after my due date but not strongly and with no regularity. When I went to bed at half past midnight I had a strong contraction. 15 minutes later another one. Then 12 minutes later, then 10 minutes, 7 minutes, 5 … It was easy to breathe through them while lying down and because I was cold I didn't want to leave my bed. I quickly got a pair of socks as I had cold feet and put child number 4 who was sleeping next to me, on the potty. My spontaneous mantra to remain relaxed during the contractions was: 'These are only powerful uterine squeezes.'

The last contraction however made me flee the bed. We had invited a film crew for this birth and they had to be called on time. When I got up, I felt shaky and my brain analysed: Transition. Am I already this far? Now everything had to be done quickly!

So I woke my husband who sorted everything: Calling the film crew, filling the water butt (in which I wanted to give birth), lighting the stove etc … Meanwhile I emptied my bladder and bowels into the toilet several times and went to the water butt.

I had my first expulsive contraction as the film crew arrived and my waters went … the baby would be there quicker than the water butt could be filled. So supported by the water butt on the left and the book case on the right I tried not to push wildly with the contractions (though the temptation was most definitely there) but attempted to breathe the baby down a la Hypnobirthing. That's what I had planned to do and it worked surprisingly well with the contractions.

Then, at 2.41am, a good 25 minutes after I shook my husband awake, our third son was born. He began to breathe as soon as his head was born and when I held him in my arms he complained noisily about his fate. The older siblings had planned to be present for the birth but they were so fast asleep that we could not wake them up. I treated myself to one thing and didn't regret it one bit: A doula for my babymoon.

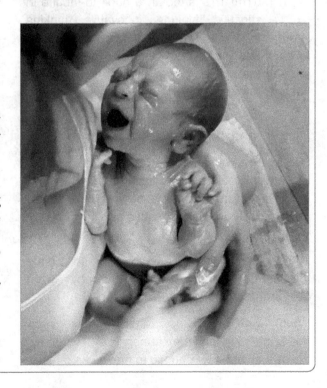

What to expect from this book

This is a very personal book. I will tell you about my thoughts and experiences and you will gain insight into other freebirthers' thoughts and experiences.

In this book you will find all the knowledge I have gained in the preparation of my own freebirths and in search of answers to other women's questions, from different sources of information.

What I wrote is also based on the experiences of other women who shared their birth stories on the internet. But I also utilised the written word and experience of birth professionals who dared to take alternative paths in obstetrics. I am mostly talking about Alfred Rockenschaub, Michel Odent, Weston Price (not a birth professional though, but a dentist with important insights on how to stay healthy naturally, even throughout pregnancy, and how to have healthy children), Gregory White, Grantly Dick-Read and Ina May Gaskin to name but a few.

Please don't expect a recipe for a dream birth! This is mostly a book to inspire instinctive thinking, innovative thinking, lateral thinking and non-conformist thinking. And to empower you to make informed decisions for yourself that come from the heart and are not influenced by fear.

It is there to help you trust your body and intuition more than all the other voices you can hear.

Don't worry: you don't need to learn this book by heart to be able to have a self-directed birth. A lot of the information in this book is there so that you can look up specific issues as and when you please.

With this book I want to give you courage to make the best decisions for you and your baby – whatever they may look like.

I don't want to exclude modern medicine from this book as it can be extremely useful when it is needed or when we choose to make use of it.

The more women are well informed about their rights, the quicker obstetrics will find its deserved place as humble servant to women and their children rather than the know-it-all guardian it is today.

In the next few chapters I devote myself to the most common questions around self-directed pregnancy and birth.

If you still have questions after reading this book, please feel free to continue to thoroughly research them to built a solid base for making informed decisions from.

About responsibility,
fear and safety

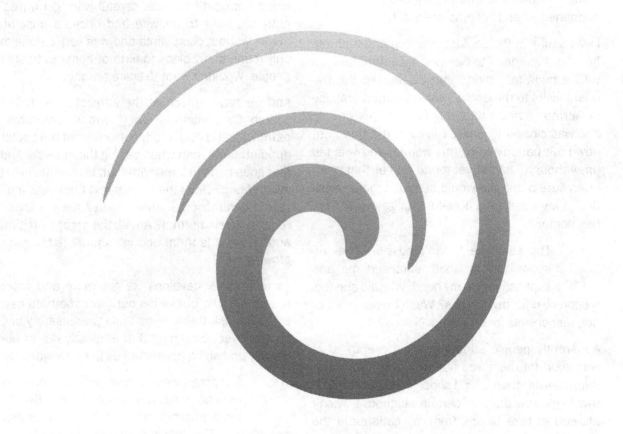

Responsibility and other people's fear

When I was holding my first positive pregnancy test just over 8 years ago, there was no question as to what I was going to do next: contact my doctor. I immediately made an appointment. I never asked myself why or indeed, if I needed to, I just did it because it is what everyone does.

'I can't possibly take responsibility for that!'

This sentence uttered by my doctor made me realise for the first time the big change that had happened when I became pregnant.

I was sitting in the doctor's practice and had told her that I intended to have all my antenatal care with a midwife. I didn't particularly like the frequent visits to the doctor (as is common practice in Germany) and I had only chosen this one as she was closest to where I lived at the time. But now I felt patronised by this woman and was fed up. Although I hadn't yet found one at that point I was sure a midwife would be much more sensitive to my needs. I just needed to get away from this doctor.

The sentence 'I can't possibly take responsibility for that!' surprised me and kept echoing in my head. Why did she feel responsible for my choices? Wasn't I, pregnant or not, responsible for my own decisions?

Apparently people suddenly knew exactly what was good for me: I was not supposed to lift anything heavier than 5 kg. I shouldn't eat raw meat, raw eggs, raw dairy or certain seafood. I wasn't allowed to take bloods from my patients in the hospital anymore or in fact get too close to them at all. I was supposed to turn up at antenatal appointments to have my blood tested and my belly examined with ultrasound. The list was endless.

No one asked me if I wanted to do all those things or if I even thought that they were necessary, but it seemed predetermined that this was best for me as a pregnant woman.

All that was expected from me was compliance. As long as I complied, everything was ok. But as soon as I declined a blood test or voiced my desire for a homebirth things became stressful.

Clearly it was not me who was responsible for my pregnancy but others: my doctor and later my midwife. Responsibility means to take the blame when something goes wrong. And no one wanted to take the blame for the misfortune of a mother and her baby.

So I did what was expected: I didn't lift heavy things (unless nobody was watching), I didn't draw any blood from patients, was careful with 'germ free' nutrition, went to midwife and doctor's appointments without complaints and was very careful to only mention my plans to birth at home to trusted people. Wouldn't want to scare anyone.

And we have arrived at the subject of fear. The search for something going wrong, something pathological is even more noticeable at the doctor appointments than when seeing the midwife. And fear goes hand in hand with that. Is the little heart still beating? Does the nuchal fold thickness indicate a chromosomal abnormality? Are the blood results etc etc normal? Are all the organs present and correct? Is there enough liquor? Is the baby growing well?

As technology develops we get more and more answers to the questions our grandmothers never had to ask themselves. It suggests safety and control over something that is mostly out of our control and still a mystery to us in many ways.

Our pregnancies are influenced in one way or another by other people's fears. But the most treacherous of all is a birth professional's fear. That fear is sometimes masked in advice or sometimes even in tasteless manipulation and threats, when the woman declines consent for certain interventions. This sometimes results in labelling the woman as irresponsible and as a danger to her baby, or calling her in her own home because she is a few days past her EDB and has declined induction or doesn't want a caesarean section despite her baby being breech.

Obstetrics often uses fear to get women to fit with the norm to alleviate the fears of society in general and not least the birth professional's. If you find yourself in front of a 'fear mongering doctor' presenting you with a worrying diagnosis, you shouldn't make any immediate decisions or give in to threats.

It is preferable to sleep on it and get a second opinion from an experienced midwife. That way one can calm down and think in peace about what might be truly the best way forward for mother and baby. Once induced or on the operating table it is too late to turn back.

Nobody can force a pregnant woman to go to even one midwife's or doctor's appointment or go to a certain hospital for birth. Every woman is free to decide for herself, although in some countries (e.g. Austria) this free decision making is penalised with a partial withdrawal of the child benefit.

Dealing with your own fears

No woman starts her pregnancy from a neutral base. Impressions around the subject of having babies are formed long before that. We think we know what a birth is like through our own birth stories told to us by our parents, our friends, people around us and last but not least the media. Somehow the fear we are surrounded with becomes our fear too.

How much trust a woman has in her own body and its ability to birth a baby can vary hugely. Someone who was born at home herself and has grown up with the attitude that birth is something positive and achievable under one's own steam is likely to be more confident than a woman whose mother didn't want any more children as her first birth was so traumatic.

When we deal with other people's fears we also need to face our own. Instinctively we try to avoid it. We are scared to face our fears. We'd rather

ignore them and find someone to take care of us and promise that everything will be all right. This is why the promises of modern obstetrics are so enticing.

It is easy to hand over responsibility. However facing your fears is necessary for a self determined birth. This means that one should neither ignore nor deny them, but look them in the eye. It is worth finding an answer to the following questions: What am I afraid of? Why am I afraid of it? How likely is it that my fear will come true? What will I do if my fear does come true? It is very valuable to answer these questions and it might even lead to the realisation that things are not as scary as originally thought.

Someone who is secure in her plans is also less influenced by external fears. For example, these days nobody would fear falling off the end of the world during a sailing trip, even if someone said that it might happen. This is because we are secure in the knowledge that the earth is round and not a disc.

To eliminate as many false expectations and insecurities I will address the very specific fears and worries that come up while thinking of a self-directed pregnancy and birth in the later chapters of this book.

For example: What are the signs by which I can tell my baby is well, without having it confirmed by a midwife or doctor? What if the cord is round the baby's neck during birth? What do I do with the cord and placenta after the birth? What if the baby gets stuck or there is a sudden emergency? For me personally, birth lost almost all of its uncertainty and unpredictability, when all those above questions and similar ones had been answered.

Women are very susceptible to specific and non specific fears in the first and last trimester of pregnancy due to the hormonal changes pregnancy brings. Even when all questions have been answered in a rational sense. In my fourth pregnancy I was still sometimes overcome with strong fear without any rhyme or reason.

I want to tell everyone who has experienced a similar thing: These fears are annoying, but they are normal and simply part of becoming a mother. It is ok to simply face them and say: 'I already know you. You are of no significance to me and you are going to be gone again soon. Until then, I can deal with you.'

It isn't always easy to deal with those fears though and I can understand how many women seek reassurance by visiting their doctor or midwife. At the same time we are such slaves to our fear that we quickly become dependent on reassurance we don't really want. With regards to self direction in pregnancy and birth, it is helpful to learn a relaxed attitude towards our fears.

In phases of my pregnancy in which I felt unsettled inside I avoided sharing my fears with people I assumed had the same fears. Everything they were likely to say would have fueled my insecurities.

This is a subject that reaches to the core of our being. It is good to feel loved, wanted and protected in this world – never mind what people say or think. A reliable sense of self is very helpful when dealing with the deepest uncertainties of humanity, and stops you drifting aimlessly.

Fear is a bad advisor, that is the saying. Whenever possible we should avoid making decisions when afraid or in a blind panic. Whatever got us worked up: It is always better to calm down and soberly assess what makes us afraid.

Usually things look less worrying once calm and usually a solution we overlooked during our initial 'fight and flight response' becomes clear.

Fear is not a bad thing per se. It can warn us of certain situations or impending danger. This is why it is important to be able to assess, validate and distinguish our fears. Are we really in danger? Is this fear irrational? What else, apart from my fear, indicates that something is wrong?

During birth, just before the pushing stage, fear plays a natural role. In this moment, hormones are released that lead to an exceptional state that can be experienced as fear. There is no actual danger but the fear is often part of the natural process that enables the woman to let go and birth her baby. This phase is generally short and is transformed into courage and determination to get the baby out when the urge to push kicks in.

Sometimes when something is actually wrong, for example a uterine rupture after a previous caesarean section, the woman does not only experience that short lived fear of transition, but continues to be scared and unsettled in combination with other signs that indicate a deviation from the normal process of birth.

To be able to assess fear during birth accurately, it is important to understand the aspects of normal birth.

The question of safety

'An obstetrician/a midwife didn't study as long as they did for nothing. You can't teach yourself everything they know. Their speciality is attending births, so you can expect them to do a good job. Why do you want to go down the difficult and risky path of doing it all yourself?'

This, or something similar is what a woman has to listen to if she doesn't want any traditional maternity care in pregnancy or during birth. It takes six years to become a doctor and to become an obstetrician and gynaecologist adds another 5 years.

A midwife will generally study for three to four years (depending on country) and has attended many births at the end of her training.

So how can someone who has got no idea decide to birth their baby without professional help?

I was lucky in that I was able to attend some births during my time in medical school before my first birth. I wasn't able to learn the best techniques or maneuvers but I could observe how babies are delivered nowadays.

I also experienced how women were bullied into inductions and caesarean sections and how they were given drugs during their births without explaining what they were and what they did. I have also met old school midwives who would physically force women to lie on their backs (most important is that the CTG records accurately), insult them (well, the baby got IN didn't it?) or perform an episiotomy despite the woman stating she doesn't want one. It was also not unusual for the midwives to push on the woman's belly with their elbows during the pushing phase.

This was just under 10 years ago. I very much hope that scenes like that are, if not completely eradicated, rare. On the whole, conditions in clinical obstetrics have improved and women are respected much more than say, 50 years ago.

However, few of the common interventions have a solid evidence base derived from solid research

with regards to effectiveness and usefulness. Quite the opposite.

These days, midwives and doctors have accepted that being upright makes birth easier. Despite that, most births in hospitals still take place in positions that make birth more difficult. Many vacuum-assisted and caesarean births could be avoided if the woman were given the chance to turn and the coccyx room to move out of the way to let the baby out.

Instead the birthing woman generally sits or lies on her coccyx (the semirecumbent position at least promises some degree of being upright but on modern delivery beds is easily transformed into the lithotomy position which means being flat on the back with legs in stirrups). Ventouse, a syntocinon drip or the Kristeller maneuver are then used when the woman predictably has difficulty birthing her baby. The Kristeller maneuver was named after the gynaecologist Samuel Kristeller and means to exert pressure on the top of the uterus during a contraction to help with expulsion of the baby.

Originally this maneuver was used to help women who had birthed several babies and therefore lacked muscle tone in their abdominals and had a diastasis recti separation (a gap between the rectus abdominis muscles). It gave the uterus resistance to push against during the expulsive phase of birth.

To use it in between contractions was considered negligent in Kristeller's times (Rockenschaub 2005). Nowadays, there thankfully aren't many women with severe diastasis recti separation as it generally develops after many pregnancies.

Despite research showing no benefits from the Kristeller maneuver, it is still being used by some birth professionals to shorten the expulsive phase of birth. (Schulz-Lobmeyr 1995)

To push against the abdominal muscles requires a certain force and it is used without hesitation. Or sometimes it is even used without a contraction, when the abdominal muscles are relaxed, entirely against the original rules. Alfred Rock-enschaub, longstanding obstetrician and former head of the Ignaz Semmelweis obstetrics and gynaecology clinic in Vienna, teacher and lecturer bluntly states what he thinks about that:

'What happens here [during use of the Kristeller maneuver] is more about violence against women than about obstetrics.' (Rockenschaub 2005)

(Note from the translator: Regarding the Kristeller maneuver there seems to be a different approach in different countries. The Kristeller maneuver is hardly ever used in the UK, except perhaps in dire emergencies and even then it is generally not regarded as acceptable... I have NEVER seen it in nearly 20 years as a midwife.)

If we look at other obstetric interventions one by one, we will find quickly that hardly any are proven to be effective. How much do the much praised and trusted obstetricians and other birth professionals really know? Do all the older women having their first, particularly big babies these days justify the rise in caesarean section rate and many other interventions?

A maternity care system with a caesarean section rate of over 30% can only be described as disastrous or amateurish. Turning it around would mean that over 30% of mothers and/or babies would have died in the olden days. But did that happen?

Not so long ago, in 1993, when the caesarean section rate in Germany was still 16.9%, maternal mortality (which is an important measure to assess quality of maternity care) accounted for 5.5 per 100.000 births. In 2001 this rate remained at 5.5 per 100.000 according to the Statistisches Bundesamt (Statistical Government Department) despite a caesarean section rate of 31.9%.

The rise in caesarean section rate is a global trend of recent years. In countries in which midwives are responsible for normal birth instead of obstetricians (France, Scandinavia) this rate is, in general, more than 10% lower than in countries in which obstetricians lead or attend births. On the whole, this trend does not have a positive impact on maternal mortality, nor on infant mortality.

Assessing maternal mortality, we have to be clear, is not an easy undertaking (due to varying definitions, limitations and difficulty collecting data) and the data we have is likely an underestimation. (Welsch 2010)

The fact that maternal mortality seems to be rising in some western countries (USA, Canada, Denmark) is also rather unsettling. In the USA, maternal morbidity has risen 42% between 1990 and 2008, despite, or perhaps because of, the high caesarean section rate. (Hogan 2010)

Are 30% of all women unable to have a normal birth despite our ingenious maternity care and highly educated birth professionals? Does the use of technology and active management of labour maybe result in less natural births? Is it possible more mothers die because of this? It seems to be that way.

To mention an example, maternal morbidity due to amniotic fluid embolism has risen considerably in the last few years. This is not surprising as it is a complication more common during caesarean sections and inductions. In 2011 for instance 8 out or 12 mothers who died did so because of an amniotic fluid embolism. (Rath 2014)

Looking at the animal kingdom is almost shocking. Ultrasound or CTG are never used except for some overbred pets. But it is not only technology cow, cat and deer do without during birth. Looking at those births from a hygiene point of view is a complete disaster. The cat gives birth to her babies on an old newspaper in a dusty corner under the sofa and the calf drops straight into a pile of manure. Cutting the cord in a sterile fashion? No chance. Cords break or are chewed off and short, bloody umbilical stumps dangle freely, open to the 'bacteria riddled' elements. Hardly any offspring should survive, thinking about it clinically.

So it is even more astonishing that deaths or extreme physical impairment due to birth is fairly rare. I grew up with rabbits and cats. Every year there was at least a litter both of cats and rabbits. Often more. Rabbits died, if at all, due to inexperienced mothers not tucking them into the warm nest or eating their young in their overeagerness to ingest the placentas.

Generally though, mothers and babies survived. And this despite the absence of professional help and mothers never attending antenatal classes. The mothers knew intuitively how to birth up to 12 babies swiftly and safely and to take them to a cosy place afterwards. All this usually happened during the night and we humans woke up to a surprise in the morning.

This poses the following question: If animals have this inborn knowledge, why shouldn't we as humans have it too? Could this instinctive knowledge also enable us humans to birth our babies safely without the need for technical-'pseudo scientific' maternity care?

Answering both questions with 'yes' leaves us wondering what exactly happened with that knowledge. Have we simply lost it in the course of history? And is it still possible for humans, guided by reason and fear, to access that knowledge and be led by intuition?

Acting intuitively means to be able to make appropriate decisions in complex situations. By listening to your gut, as the saying goes. Obviously humans still have this innate, subconscious knowledge, our intuition.

Here is a typical story that I have heard again and again which illustrates the issue of intuition beautifully.

' I had really wanted a homebirth for my first baby, I felt deep inside that I would just want to go into our bathroom and stay there all by myself. But then external pressure was stronger than my desire and the common belief that hospital is best took over. This is how my imagined freebirth became a caesarean section as I found out too late that I cannot give birth in front of an audience. After a pre labour rupture of membranes and an attempt

to induce me via syntocinon drip in the hospital, I started having strong intestinal cramping and the birth stalled. Instead of leaving me in peace for a while, it was thought more syntocinon would help but it only led to the baby not wanting to be born at all. I felt utterly powerless and insecure in that situation and it took me years to accept the caesarean section and to recognise my mistakes. Luckily I trusted my intuition for the following two births and stayed at home. I was attended by a midwife for my second birth and wanted to take the birth into my own hands and planned a freebirth with only the baby and I for my third birth.' (Caroline, mother of three daughters)

Ignoring your intuition is easily done if the voices around us are loud and intrusive. Sometimes those voices force themselves on us by making us scared.

Scared that something bad could happen if we trust our inner voice, scared not to fit in with societal norms and being judged. Scared to disappoint people. Scared not to be loved anymore because of our choices. Scared we might be intrinsically wrong and fall flat on our faces, with a baby on board, no less. However, this intrinsic knowledge we don't know the exact origin of, called intuition, is a very powerful tool indeed. We gain knowledge about the everyday things in life in school, university, though books, the internet and countless other sources.

But only intuition helps us put our knowledge into context in any given scenario. It helps us decide what to do in certain situations and what is best for us. Ideally, intuition works hand in hand with the knowledge we already have. It makes us more decisive in our decision-making, without having to think too much.

To be able to use intuition as a reliable tool for our decision-making in birth, we have to practice. We have to learn to recognise its voice and trust it. What time better for this than the nine months of pregnancy?

During pregnancy every woman can practice listening to her inner voice:

- What do I need?
- What do I want?
- What has positive or negative effect on my well being?
- Are my baby's movements really reduced or is he well and just a little sleepy?
- Are these harmless Braxton-Hicks contractions or do I have reason to worry?

Waiting and coping with uncertainty is not easy. But at the end of the day, we can be certain about what we really want.

During my first unassisted pregnancy I was unsure when to or indeed if I should see a midwife after all. First I picked a certain week of my pregnancy as my personal boundary, but moved it further and further along as I felt uncomfortable with the thought of being measured and judged.

At the same time I was unsure as I had chosen a path nobody else seemed to be considering. Was I mad and would soon pay for my recklessness? Was the positive feeling I had for myself and my lively baby perhaps deceiving me?

Making an appointment with the midwife would have removed this feeling of uncertainty, yet it would have manoeuvered me into a situation I didn't want to be in. I coped with the uncertainty in the knowledge that most women in the history of mankind, like me, had been pregnant and birthed healthy babies easily.

'But hold on!' some will interrupt me. 'Weren't maternal and newborn mortality rates much higher in those days? Don't mothers and babies still die much more frequently in Africa? We should be pleased and thankful for the blessing that is modern medicine!'

In some aspects modern medicine certainly is a blessing. But there are things that are more important with regards to a safe birth than medical care: clean drinking water, enough food, the absence of war and unrest and a warm, dry place to live. The more a country lacks those conditions, the more frequently do births end in complications and death, and perhaps then more modern medicine – as well as other things – is required for damage limitation.

To compare the quality of maternity care in different countries, we can use maternal mortality rates, as already mentioned. Those are defined by the WHO as follows:

'Maternal death is the death of a woman while pregnant or within 42 days of termination of pregnancy, irrespective of the duration and site of the pregnancy, from any cause related to or aggravated by the pregnancy or its management but not from accidental or incidental causes (whose accident or incident we are talking about is not defined, added by author)' (World Health Organisation WHO)

Causes of maternal death vary worldwide, but the majority are due to poverty, war, malnutrition, and lack of medical care. Many women die from haemorrhage after botched abortions, which has a big impact on maternal death statistics.

The poorer the country and living conditions, the higher the mother and infant mortality. While only one in 3800 mothers dies in industrial nations, the rate shoots up to one in 39 mothers in sub saharan Africa. 99% of all maternal deaths take place in developing countries at this point in time. (German Foundation for World Population 2012)

Europe also had a high mortality rate for mothers and newborns during the middle ages and the early 20th century. German birthing homes had particularly high rates as doctors taught their medical students clinical obstetrics with the help of the destitute women forced to use them. The women's confinements often ended in death if the doctors or students had also dissected dead bodies as part of their studies.

It only became possible to birth in hospitals without the imminent threat of death, when doctors learned about bacteria, antibiotics and hygiene measures to keep mothers safe. Unfortunately we lack data from earlier periods or civilisations to speculate about the history of obstetrics.

We do however have lots of anecdotal reports from explorers and anthropologists (predominantly from the first half of the 20th century) and those overwhelmingly mention quick and uncomplicated births.

Today, maternal mortality is very low comparatively, mostly due to good living conditions but also generally more knowledge and modern medicine. Birthplace, either home or hospital doesn't seem to play a role.

Studies regarding the safety of midwife attended homebirths after an uncomplicated pregnancy show that homebirths are as safe as hospital births (4.3 adverse outcomes in 1000 birth regardless of place of birth), at the same time homebirths show the advantage of less interventions and birth trauma (Brocklehurst 2011). From interviewing women we also know that overall subjective satisfaction is greater for women who birthed their babies at home. (Eirich 2012)

How about homebirths without a midwife though? A mostly prospective study of 400 planned freebirths including twins showed the following outcomes: 88% of the births were successful freebirths. A change from the original plan of freebirth happened in 12% of cases. 10.8% transferred into hospital, just about 1.3% consulted a midwife and 3.3% ended in a caesarean section. There were no maternal or infant deaths associated with the births (Hessel 2008).

This study originated from the USA where midwifery care is much less common. The hospital transfer rate would likely have been lower in most European countries as more midwives would have been consulted to attend women at home. However, this much is true: It can only show us the average outcome. It doesn't tell us how the birth went for each individual woman, which, at the end of the day, is the only thing that counts.

Luckily we are not victims of chance getting sorted into our little statistical niche, but we can purposefully work towards a safe, healthy birth without hospital, monitoring and even a midwife.

A first time mother doesn't tend to have experience of a normal birth unless she is a midwife, but that can be of advantage. A midwife might bring fears into the birth that lead her to call off her freebirth earlier than a mother well prepared for freebirth.

When planning a birth without a midwife it is a good idea to cover your back in two different ways. Knowledge of basic obstetrics paired with good old intuition gives us double reassurance. If women have intuitive knowledge about birth, just like animals, we can assume that, with basic knowledge of obstetrics, they may be just as effective as a midwife or even better at determining what to do in any given situation.

When it comes to ideal birthing position, the right time to start pushing, stimulating a less than lively newborn or the decision to transfer to hospital: many women's experiences show that a carefully prepared freebirth can be very successful in all those aspects.

I'm often told 'You were just lucky!' Sometimes I can almost hear regret that nothing went wrong and I didn't get comeuppance for my 'irresponsibility'. It is easy to see that my preparations were extensive. Not only from an intellectual point of view, but also physically (nutrition, exercise) and spiritually (working through fears, surrounding myself with lovely things, visualising the birth).

When a pregnant woman decides to take the birth into her own hands, she doesn't act thoughtlessly just hoping for a lucky twist of fate. What looks like luck to others is really a natural chain of events in a process that is innate to us women, and often it happens even without any preparations as shown by many accidental and unplanned freebirths, that unfolded without fear or disturbance.

As you can see from the birth stories in the second part of the book however, some planned freebirths do end with a transfer into hospital and some even with a caesarean section. Although this is generally, as I have been able to glean from all the birth stories I have read so far, an astonishingly small minority of all freebirthers.

Can we therefore assume with good conscience that all will be well? Generally, yes, as we can see looking at the world's population. It doesn't matter if you believe in evolution or creationism, it would be illogical if birth of all things was a process not designed to be successful. So the only question is, what can we do to keep this process, which is individual to all women and their babies, undisturbed?

But what about babies who die during birth? There will always be stories of loss. Not even the best technology and the strictest monitoring in hospitals can eliminate those. And looking at modern obstetrics, it seems that in its eagerness to make birth 100% safe it has gone the other way and caused more damage than positive outcomes in many cases.

Why? Firstly, because medical knowledge evolves constantly, quicker than ever nowadays. It is not set in stone for all eternity, far from it. Also, our own interpretation of history is subjective and influenced by our experience and thoughts. In this sense, the chasm between knowledge and intuition is smaller than we thought. Errors and relative truths exist on both sides and usually we get the best outcome by bringing both sides together.

Doctors of course deserve respect for their knowledge and experience, but we have to remember that even they are influenced by their own fears and experiences. Even if a doctor is very experienced in attending births in a hospital setting, he will likely see himself in the context of hospital routines and the experiences he had in this setting. He will lack knowledge about a mother's intuition and fully physiological, natural births. Medical advice can reflect hospital guidelines and the newest research findings, yet still not be appropriate for the birthing woman. This is why we shouldn't take any advice as absolute truth and rather listen to our intuition and get a second opinion from a trusted person.

Is midwifery care the best alternative to medical care? The knowledge and experience of a longstanding homebirth midwife can be invaluable, especially if the chemistry between mother and midwife is right. She can be especially helpful for a first time mother and, hopefully with absolute positivity and trust, help remove potential insecurities. Despite that, pregnant women should be aware that not everything the midwife may advise is right for them and, as already mentioned, even a midwife can bring fears to the table that really shouldn't be taken on board without further research.

The description of freebirth often suggests that the birthing woman is alone and completely left to her own devices, but this is generally rare and at least the woman's partner is in attendance. What role exactly family support may play and how it is possible to respect womens' autonomy without influencing her with fear, can be found onwards from page 115.

Nutrition as key for healthy pregnancy and birth

The recipe for success from ancient civilisations

Nutrition is one of the building blocks that helps create the basis for a healthy pregnancy and birth in which a doctor is not needed.

Though what actually makes for a healthy diet is not so easy to determine these days. Research findings and interpretations vary greatly and accordingly, recommendations are ten a penny.

Despite lacking our up-to-date knowledge and research many civilisations have lived in amazingly good health. Life expectancy was often short due to harsh living conditions, but even though many more people died from accidents and conflict, many others lived to a ripe old age of around 70. (Gurven 2007)

An obvious decline in health only happened when western diet and habits took over (Price 2010). This is why I feel that nutrition like that of our early ancestors makes the most sense.

Until the first half of the 20th century many explorers visited indigenous tribes, that mostly lived without contact with western civilisation and were still fairly common in those days. The explorers were amazed that common diseases were almost unheard of in their culture. Amongst them were: cancer, arthritis, asthma, dental caries, dental malocclusion, shortsightedness and a whole host of other degenerative, inflammatory diseases (Berglas 1957). They were equally amazed as to how quickly and effortlessly women gave birth to their babies (Price 2010).

One of those explorers was dentist and nutritionist Weston Price (1870–1948). He analysed the health of the indigenous people he visited and the nutritional value of their food and found that they consumed at least four times more calcium and ten times more fat soluble vitamins than the average American person.

Based on Price's findings and those of his contemporaries we can make valuable recommendations regarding nutrition that not only benefit pregnant women but also the population in general.

Rule 1: Sugar: very little and natural

In preindustrial times, sweet things were much desired yet rare. Our high sugar consumption plays a large, if not deciding part in the development of many modern diseases, like dental caries, most types of cancer (Quillin 2005) and diabetes as well as in the trend towards obesity. Instead of fat making us ill and fat, as is traditionally believed, it is the constant blood sugar spikes due to our high sugar consumption.

To keep blood sugar levels as even as possible under these conditions, our body constantly pushes sugar into its cells where it is laid down as fat. A high sugar consumption also changes vaginal bacterial flora, making vaginal infections more likely which in turn increases the risk of premature birth.

This change in bacterial flora can also be responsible for digestive disorders as well as autoimmune and chronic inflammatory diseases (Brown 2012).

The food industry adds sugar to virtually everything, and many people literally have withdrawal symptoms when eliminating sugar for a day. Giving up sugar is possible though.

Cutting out processed foods, establishing new habits and replacing sugar with good quality fats and protein is the way to do it. If the body still craves sugar after a couple of weeks withdrawing from sugar, a different important nutrient might be the culprit for those cravings.

Rule 2: Carefully prepared grains

Cultures that heavily relied on grains as their staple food spent a lot of time preparing those grains appropriately by sprouting, drying, grinding, sieving and fermenting. This produced a healthful product, even if consumed regularly.

Time is of the essence in our modern society however and therefore those practices have largely disappeared. People who want to eat healthily often count on whole grains and dietary fibre while overlooking that most of the vitamins and minerals in whole grains are tied to phytic acid (a so called antinutrient) and therefore are not bioavailable to our bodies without careful preparation.

This phytic acid is predominantly found in the outer hull of grains and protects the kernel from mould and pests but hinders absorption of nutrients by the body.

It is optimal to take the middle path when it comes to the consumption of grains as is the case in traditional societies. The outer hull of the grain is removed, but not so completely as to be left with white flour. This is how much of the nutrients are preserved. Fermenting then removes many of the antinutrients present in the grain. (Urbano 2000)

In addition to that a diet high in fat soluble vitamins largely neutralises the effect of any remaining antinutrients (Mellanby 1949). Sourdough bread is an example of traditional grain processing that has found its way into present times.

Rule 3: The whole animal is edible

Going to the shops we generally see chicken breast, perhaps legs and wings in the cooler. But where are the other parts of the chicken: neck, head, feet, bones, blood and giblets?

Organ meats especially are very rich in vitamins and minerals. Blood has lots of iron. Bones make beautiful broth that is superior both in flavour and quality to any stock cube (made from salt, flavour enhancers, vegetable oils and sugar).

Traditional societies valued and found use for every part of the animal, including the intestine, sometimes even including the contents. With rising prosperity, meals made from organ meats have gained the label of 'poor people's food' and have mostly been forgotten. We are missing out on the most vitamin and mineral dense cuts of meat. But because our way of eating is traditional to us, we don't realise that there is something not quite right with our diet.

The trend towards vegetarianism and veganism is also not reflected in human history so far. Apart from the odd cultural shunning of meat for religious reasons, all civilisations have made good use of meat, fat, dairy and co.

Rule 4: Fat is best

Muscle meat was not considered the best cut of meat in the olden days. American Indians much preferred shooting an old, fat buffalo, than a lean young one and their dietary intake nearly reached 80% fat on occasion. (Stefansson 1960)

Traditionally, fat was best in all cultures. They obviously lacked scientific background as to why, but because it was tasty and kept them full, they favoured animal fat. And they kept themselves healthy eating this diet, because: fat contains all those extremely important fat soluble vitamins (Vitamin D,A,K and E) that we often lack in our low fat diet. Due to that we increasingly suffer from caries, depression, osteoporosis or skin and connective tissue disorders, to name but a few.

Meanwhile we have accumulated plenty of studies showing that saturated fat is not directly connected with our lifestyle diseases (Ravnskov 2010). That would indeed be absurd as traditional cultures used to ingest (and still do) far more saturated fat than we do without suffering from our modern diseases. Furthermore it is now known that the body itself produces most of its own cholesterol. Eating less only results in the body making more of it.

These days, research on fat has moved away from the hypothesis that 'saturated fats make us fat and sick'. Furring up arteries with plaques requires an inflammatory process in the body (Tousoulis 2006) but finding the cause for that is a multilayered scientific question we have yet to answer.

In this context it is probably appropriate to mention that refined vegetable oils such as rapeseed and sunflower oil are not found in the diet of any indigenous cultures and due to their manufacturing process raise concerns about their healthfulness. Their polyunsaturated fatty acids are not heat stable and change in the manufacturing process of which heating is only a small part.

These altered fatty acids ('transfats') especially, along with sugar, are suspected in playing a large part in causing inflammatory processes in the body that in turn lead to our modern diseases. (Mozaffarian 2004 & 2006, Karbowska 2011)

Harmless however are cold pressed vegetable oils (they should not be heated to high temperatures though) and fats and oils consisting of mostly saturated and monounsaturated fatty acids, such as butter, lard, olive or coconut oil. The latter (saturated and monounsaturated) fats and oils can withstand high cooking temperatures without changing their structure and are ideal for frying and cooking.

Rule 5: Dirt is not the enemy

The German saying 'Dirt cleanses the stomach.' is not altogether wrong.

Research has established that a person who was exposed to dirt and bacteria in childhood, for example like the ones commonly found on a farm, has a lower chance of developing allergies and asthma. (Lauener 2002)

When going abroad to places such as India, it is common knowledge to avoid buying foods from street vendors and to wash fruit and vegetables thoroughly to avoid 'Monezuma's revenge', meaning diarrhea. Interestingly, this terrible diarrhea does not normally affect any locals. Their immune system is clearly accustomed to the bacteria we worry about and they rarely suffer from allergies.

In the western world we are big on hygiene and taught that a lack of bacteria equals health. Therefore we clean, heat and pasteurise liberally.

As well as bacteria we also destroy living cells present in our food and much of its vitamin and enzyme content. We end up asking ourselves why our immune systems are running amok and can't tolerate many of the devitalised products we consume.

Nowadays we hardly ever consume all those bacteria which were commonly found in foods in the olden days. Then, fruits and vegetables were fertilised with manure, not with man made chemicals as is the case now. We drank raw milk and soured milk products were not made with industrially made bacteria but contained a variety of natural bacterial cultures. This is how we consumed healthy bacteria on a day to day basis.

But we know: The more variety in the bacteria of the gut flora, the better our digestive as well as immune function. Suboptimal bacterial population of the gut makes us more likely to develop food intolerances, allergies, autoimmune diseases and even depression and other mental health issues. (Bercik 2011)

Our fear of listeria, toxoplasmosis and co and our avoidance of raw foods in pregnancy makes us forget not only that those diseases are extremely rare but also that there is another component to consider: our immune system.

A robust immune system is likely to stay that way in pregnancy and it's worth testing boundaries before pregnancy and injecting a healthy dose of microorganisms into our diet.

Rule 6: Sauerkraut as medicine

In the time before fridges and pickling jars we had to find other methods to preserve our foods. Most cultures used fermentation, also called souring or lactofermentation, to keep foods from spoiling and make them more digestible.

Sauerkraut is the most well known of all fermented foods. Eating it fresh and not from a jar from the supermarket provides us with a good amount of healthy bacteria and vitamins beneficial for digestion.

Other fermented foods include yogurt, quark, buttermilk, kefir, sourdough, sour pickled vegetables, kombucha (fermented green tea) or korean kimchi.

Rule 7: Daily consumption of raw milk

Traditionally, milk was never heat pasteurised. Not even 100 years ago milk around the world was always consumed raw. When it turned sour, people would drink soured milk or it was made into quark or cheese.

In the era of industrialisation however, raw milk became a health hazard. For the first time cows were kept in massive dairy farms and were provided with food very differently to what they would naturally eat out in the grassy pastures. Not only did the quality of milk decline, the cows' health did too.

Science had a solution though: Pasteurisation. Yes, taste suffered, but pasteurisation was written into law in the name of health anyway.

Milk's reputation has taken a hit due to speculation about dairy being part responsible for many of our lifestyle diseases. But looking at the fact that those diseases are relatively new to us as a population, as well as pasteurisation, it makes sense to come to the conclusion that raw grassfed dairy is not the problem. Perhaps there is a problem with our homogenised,

pasteurised, artificially preserved milk. Due to better hygiene and lifestock nutrition, raw milk nowadays is very different to the raw milk of 100 years ago when it often contributed to the spread of diseases like tuberculosis.

Feeding lifestock corn silage, as is common nowadays, is of course far from species appropriate, but it was even less appropriate in those days. It was not uncommon to feed dairy cattle with plant based waste products left over from brewing, sawdust or other waste from industrial processes. (Sherrard 1920, Reif 1996)

A review of the studies available today shows that raw milk does not pose a health risk nowadays (Ijaz 2013) but it might take quite some time until this is reflected in official recommendations.

Women who are able to access raw milk from mostly hay or grass fed cattle and who have a reasonably robust immune system should not have to worry about enjoying raw milk, even in pregnancy.

Another advantage of untreated milk, apart from its high vitamin and healthy bacteria content, is the fact that many people unable to digest pasteurised milk can actually drink it without encountering problems.

Rule 8: Particular foods that prepare for pregnancy

In his book 'Nutrition and Physical degeneration' Weston Price mentions the careful preparation for pregnancy in traditional cultures.

Not only were pregnancies timed carefully so babies were born at certain times of the year or with sufficient gap between siblings but pregnant women were also given particular foods in preparation for and during pregnancy such as roe, shrimp or the ash of certain plants. This was to secure a healthy, well developed offspring. (Price 2010)

Such traditional knowledge has largely disappeared. It has been replaced by modern medicine and blanket recommendations regarding iodine (in Germany) and folic acid supplementation and fruit and vegetable intake.

This however does not seem to be adequate substitution for the nutrient dense particular foods recommended by ancient civilisations.

Important vitamins and minerals for pregnancy and breastfeeding

If you feel you might be deficient in one or more of the following nutrients, try to supplement your diet with natural foods or supplements rather than artificially manufactured ones that often cannot be absorbed as readily as their more natural counterpart or might even be harmful.

Calcium and Vitamin D

Both of these are necessary for bone and tooth development in the fetus. Vitamin D helps the body utilise calcium.

A good balance of calcium and vitamin D can protect the pregnant woman from raised blood pressure and preeclampsia (Ramos 2006), as well as contribute to a quick painless birth as some authors claim (Davis 1972, Kitzinger 2002).

Signs of calcium deficiency are dry skin, caries, brittle bones, tingly hands and feet and leg cramps. Oxalic acid (e.g in spinach) and phytic acid (in unfermented grains, beans, nuts and seeds) inhibits calcium absorption.

Foods rich in calcium are milk and dairy products, bone broth, leafy green vegetables and herbs (such as nettles and dandelion). Vitamin D is found in cod liver oil, oily fish, egg yolk, animal fats and whole milk.

Magnesium

Lack of magnesium can show itself through pregnancy sickness in the first trimester (Latva-Pukkila 2010), cramp (Dahle 1995, Supakatisant 2012), recurrent miscarriages (Seelig 1980), premature labour, low birth weight (Makrides 2012) and preeclampsia (Standley 1997, Witlin 1998, Azria 2004).

Foods high in magnesium are: cocoa, bone broth, wholemeal products (please use sourdough though, as the phytic acid in the grain bonds to the magnesium otherwise, making it very hard to absorb), roasted pumpkin seeds, sunflower seeds, cashew nuts, almonds, beans, spinach and other green vegetable, halibut, mackerel and mineral water. The body needs Vitamin B6, B12 and calcium to be able to utilise magnesium.

Iron

It is normal for iron levels to drop below usual levels in pregnancy. In fact, the drop seems to convey some protection against infections. (Weiss 2009)

Iron supplements should really only be taken if a low iron level has been diagnosed reliably and goes hand in hand with associated symptoms (tiredness, hair loss, pallor, headaches). It is important to realise that low iron levels are often coupled with folic acid and vitamin B12 deficiency.

Food with high levels of iron are liver (pork, beef), black pudding, lentils, oysters, chanterelle mushrooms. Many women find supplementing with herbal elixirs available in health food shops very helpful.

Zinc

Susceptibility to infections, fungal diseases and stretch marks can be a sign of zinc deficiency in pregnancy. (Watts 1988, Stamm 2009)

Even severe pregnancy sickness is associated with a lack of zinc. (Latva-Pukkila 2010)

Good sources of zinc are oysters, beef, pork and calves liver, cheese and beef, nuts and beans.

Zinc deficiency can also result from raised copper levels in the blood (for example due to water from copper pipes) and excessively high iron levels (due to iron supplementation) because zinc, copper and iron compete for the same medium of transport in the blood.

Vitamin B6

Vitamin B6 deficiency stands in connection with raised insulin resistance as well as oxidative stress (Shen 2010), severe pregnancy nausea, decreased fertility and a higher rate of miscarriages. (Matthews 2010, Ronnenberg 2007)

A severe deficiency may result in skin rashes on the head, anaemia, and numb or painful hands and feet.

Organ meats like beef liver and kidney, beef, pork, poultry, mackerel, sardines, potatoes, cabbage, avocado and bananas are especially rich in vitamin B6.

Wholegrain foods and other plant sources also contain vitamin B6 but the vitamin is more bioavailable from animal sources.

Vitamin B12

Vitamin B12 deficiency results in anaemia, difficulty sleeping, depression and neurological illness.

It is also associated with a higher risk of neural tube defects in the fetus, such as spina bifida and anencephaly (absence of a major portion of the brain) as well as delayed motor and psychological development in utero and in infancy and abnormal blood values. (Molloy 2009, Kühne 1991, Dror 2008)

Generally though the signs of B12 deficiency are rather non-specific. It is also difficult to diagnose via a blood serum test for B12. A diagnosis is more reliable when measuring methylmalonic acid levels and holotranscobalamin. (Hermann 2008)

B12 is found mostly in animal derived sources. In adults, B12 stores usually last for several years so that a deficiency only becomes apparent after eating a suboptimal diet for a long time. Children however have only had time to build up very small stores.

Vegans, especially in pregnancy, should carefully supplement their diet with vitamin B12. (Koebnick 2004)

Folic Acid

Folic acid is another nutrient that stands in connection with neural tube defects as well as with cardiac abnormalities (Czeizel 2013). There also seems to be a connection with a higher incidence of miscarriages. (Ronnenberg 2002)

The anaemia that results from being deficient in folic acid leads to tiredness, pallor, depression and palpitations. Other symptoms include diarrhoea and digestive problems. However, all these fairly non specific indicators can have entirely different causes (often multiple deficiencies are to blame) and should absolutely be taken seriously.

Foods high in folic acid include wheatgerm, kidney beans, kale, spinach, other leafy green vegetables, calves' liver, yeast and eggs.

Practical Pregnancy

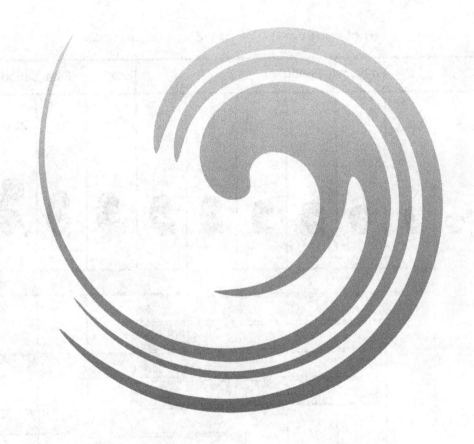

Pregnant?

Congratulations! You are pregnant!

A tiny little speck of life has started to grow inside you. With breathtaking speed it will turn into a tiny baby to hold in your arms and nurture at your breast. How amazing!

No scientist in the world can replicate what you are doing without even consciously trying. It doesn't matter if you are asleep or awake, your body is growing your baby all by itself.

The following graphic shows how your baby develops during each week of pregnancy.

The light grey areas depict the time period in which the structural basis of each particular body part is laid down.

The dark grey area shows the time period in which the development concludes, and after which time only growth with regards to size and weight takes place.

What happens in the weeks of pregnancy?

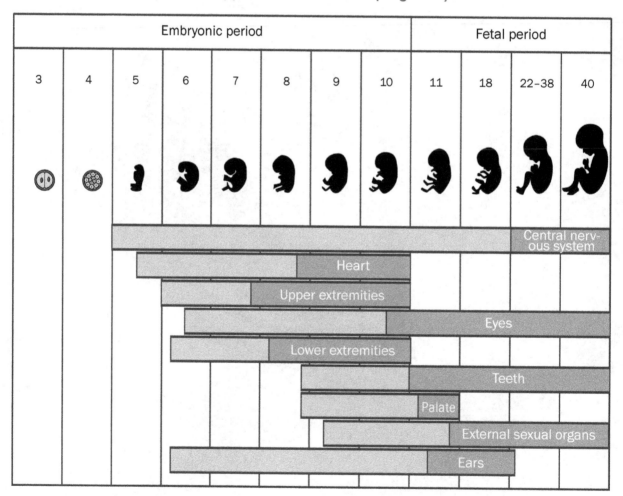

About moods and sensitivities

From now on you will spend a lot of time thinking about the tiny human inside you, and that is how it should be.

Maybe this baby is the result of trying to get pregnant for a long time. Maybe you had already given up hope. Maybe this pregnancy is entirely unexpected. Maybe you have previously lost a baby or had a termination. Maybe you are already taking care of a whole brood of offspring and you are worried that it is all going to get too much.

Whatever feelings you are experiencing now: your baby is a gift. Even when you are not rejoicing with excitement right now, one day he will bring you joy.

So now you know you are pregnant. I bet you already know what is expected of you as your next step. But you are not quite sure what is good and necessary for yourself in this pregnancy. Or you might know exactly what you will need but are not quite sure how to go about actually getting it. And already you are busy making plans. Do you have a name? How will the birth be? What will it be like with a new baby in the house?

Pregnancy brings many physical and emotional changes. Mostly responsible are your changing hormone levels and there is precious little you can do. Suddenly opening up the spice cabinet makes you throw up. Maybe you feel so sick that you are hardly managing to eat. You might all of a sudden fancy odd food combinations or feel so tired that you fall asleep in the middle of the day.

You could just start crying whenever babies are mentioned. Rudeness from other people really starts getting to you and you just want to isolate yourself from all the bad things in the world, even if previously you were a very outgoing person who never flinched away from any unpleasantness.

Your partner seems really insensitive now and you are constantly bickering. You always feel like you are absolutely in the right and when your partner comes out with things like 'You are obnoxious when you are pregnant.' or similar, you are even more enraged and feel like no one takes you seriously. Hopefully they will be understanding because pregnancy lasts quite a while.

It is not unlikely that you might also start to feel conflicted about your antenatal care. Maybe you had originally planned to go to all your appointments and now you don't want others to intrude into your happy pregnancy bubble.

Perhaps you didn't want ultrasound scans at all in this pregnancy, but in the weeks of waiting for the baby's first movements you felt worried and switched on the baby TV after all.

You will probably find that your emotions are all over the place, particularly towards the beginning and the end of pregnancy. Give in to the changes you are going through, accept the uncertainties and surround yourself with positivity. If your family is stressing you out, talk to them or reduce contact. If your doctor is annoying you, go to a different one, your midwife or neither.

Do what makes you feel good. Nap, give in to your cravings (but be careful with regards to sugar), surround yourself with positivity and enjoy your growing belly (despite potential discomforts). Talk to your unborn baby! It will bond you and in a certain way your baby can already understand you.

Dear mother, you are beautiful with your belly and your soft curves. What is happening inside you is as ordinary as it could possibly be but yet it is miraculous. You are growing life and will birth a tiny new human. Enjoy it. You are carrying a miracle and are miraculous yourself.

The best care

Established antenatal care offered by doctors and midwives is fairly similar in western countries. Protocol generally determines what sort of tests are offered and when. This rarely takes into account individual need but rather concerns itself with prevention and early treatment of pregnancy complications for mother and baby, preferably in a time and cost effective manner of course.

Women usually do not get consulted as to whether they are happy to have all the care offered or if the care is indeed appropriate for them as individuals. Unless they specifically decline, the predetermined protocol will be followed.

A midwife has a little more time and inclination to determine individual wishes and needs, but still has to follow protocol and work in a cost and time efficient manner.

 To figure out which model of care may be best for you, it makes sense to think about what you are expecting:

- Do you want results from certain laboratory tests to put your mind at rest?
- Do you have any pre-existing conditions that require you to have certain investigations?
- Do you want ultrasound images for the photo album?
- Or do you feel that you mostly need someone to talk to and who can allay your fears?

While a doctor is on the medical side of the spectrum and is very much able to order certain tests and assess abnormal findings, a midwife is more in the middle of the spectrum. On the opposite end, a friend who has given birth herself or a doula may satisfy all your needs.

What sort of care each individual woman needs or wants varies widely. But is it possible to decline all formal care and still know with certainty that all is well?

The answer is: yes, essentially it is possible and it certainly is not illegal. Many women who plan to birth without an attendant also have a self-directed pregnancy.

In my last four pregnancies I didn't see any doctors or midwives and didn't have any medical tests for myself or my baby. For me, this was best.

It was clear to me: as long as I am only pregnant and not sick, I don't want to be assessed.

Other women might cherry pick a few tests they feel are valuable but decline others. Basically: if you don't strictly follow protocol, you have plenty of freedom to create your very own custom package of care for your pregnancy.

Of course babies don't need any investigations to realise they need to grow. But many women find listening to their baby's heartbeat very reassuring. Some women who do their antenatal care themselves, regularly take their own blood pressure or weigh themselves, as a midwife or doctor would do. It is also possible to check vaginal pH levels to detect signs of infection and therefore risk of premature birth.

In my first self-directed pregnancy I imitated a lot of conventional antenatal care. This became less and less with each pregnancy as my self-confidence grew and I had to battle fewer fears. Physically I was very aware of my body and I knew everything was all right, even without taking any measurements.

Finding a good midwife

Experienced midwives will always play a big role in pregnancy and birth for most women, despite the potential for self-direction. Particularly during a first pregnancy, anxiety often reigns and women find midwifery care encouraging and helpful.

Many freebirthers find it reassuring to have a midwife as back up who they can call on should doubts arise or perhaps after the birth. Even if pregnancy and birth happen without midwifery help, it is practical to have a midwife who is willing to sign documents to make registering the birth easier (it seems that for parents, registering a birth without a professional signature may be easier in Austria and Switzerland than in some areas in Germany).

However, it is not necessarily easy to find the right midwife. For many women it is difficult to find a midwife who is supportive of plans to birth at home or comfortable to be back up for a free-birth. Searching the internet as well as chatting to women with home and freebirth experience can be invaluable in locating someone sympathetic towards your plans. Sometimes widening the search radius can be worthwhile and starting to look earlier rather than later in pregnancy, before 20–24 weeks, is best.

How do I recognise a good midwife? If you are looking for a homebirth midwife, choose carefully, presuming of course that you have a choice.

The chemistry between you has to be right. But don't be deterred by a midwife's surly nature. Oftentimes midwives like that are the peace in the midst of your storm and solid as a rock during birth. Others who are always smiley and happy are sometimes not the most confident and tend to be more anxious during labour, potentially with a lower threshold for transfer to hospital.

I don't mean to tell you which type of midwife to go for obviously, I just wanted to point out that it doesn't always pay off to decide on the basis of either being a bit surly or particularly smiley. Ask lots of questions, listen carefully and ask women who have used the midwives you are thinking about using. You have a right to criticize and to articulate your wishes. These are some things to find out:

- Is the midwife experienced in homebirth, even in special circumstances such as VBAC?
- Under which circumstances would she recommend transfer?
- Does she attend breech births?

- What is her protocol regarding longer pregnancies?
- Does she insist on certain tests (for example scans, Group B Strep)?
- What happens if things deviate from the norm, like slightly elevated blood pressure?
- Would she wait in the next room if the woman wishes to be alone during birth?
- Is she happy to attend births without doing any vaginal examinations?
- Is she happy for women to catch their own babies?
- Does she agree with the concept of freebirth?

All those important questions should have been answered before a decision regarding the choice of midwife is made, but even then you can have unpleasant surprises. I know a woman who had discussed all these questions with her midwife and was all set for her homebirth when her midwife got cold feet 12 days over her estimated date of birth. The midwife claimed she didn't have a good feeling about the situation anymore and referred the woman to the hospital. The woman decided otherwise and birthed alone.

Another woman who was planning a homebirth had a midwife who insisted on ultrasound scans during which abnormalities in the baby's lungs were found. Many scans followed as well as many other tests and close antenatal surveillance. Homebirth was out. The baby was eventually born in hospital, fit as a fiddle.

I could go on with the list of unpleasant surprises. It shows us that midwives are only human. They often have lots of experience and great instincts but can also be wrong. Everyone needs to be aware of that and not simply hand over responsibility, as tempting as it might be.

Doula, friend, partner – different considerations about your birth partner

A doula is a woman who generally has had children herself and who supports women during birth in a protective helper role. Doulas can be found via the internet nowadays.

Perhaps you have a good friend who has had a self-directed birth and who is willing to help! A doula or friend can come to the birth as an addition to a midwife and attend to the needs of the labouring mother.

Some women don't have a midwife at all and only have a doula, friend or their partner around during birth. There are men who are naturals as birth partners but some would be better off going to the cinema or playground with any older children. With that in mind, a man who is generally relaxed and calm in life is likely able to remain so in other unpredictable situations, unlike a man who is of a nervous disposition.

Women know their men best and can make appropriate plans during pregnancy.

Listen to your gut when choosing the right midwife and/or doula. Birth is an exceptional situation that is likely going to test your strength and you shouldn't have to waste any of that on managing the people around you.

When you need an obstetrician

During a healthy pregnancy a healthy woman does not need a doctor, or in fact any other professional, to confirm what she already knows.

But not all women have a body that works impeccably and not every pregnancy runs its course without problems.

In those cases a good, thoughtful obstetrician is worth their weight in gold. Nowadays most obstetricians are quite convinced that homebirth is a very irresponsible undertaking. Most have not dealt with homebirthing women unless they have been transferred into hospital. Obstetricians are also the ones who deliver over 30% of babies by caesarean section in Germany, the USA, Switzerland and several other countries. Their practice generally teaches them that, in the majority of cases, birth needs some sort of intervention. With this experience, day in and day out, it is understandable they feel their intervention saves countless lives and women are almost unable to birth a baby without medical help.

Seeing that midwives and doctors are in some sense still in conflict, it is no surprise that obstetricians often feel negatively towards homebirth.

Doctors who closely work with midwives are often more open towards birthing at home. But this much is still true: don't hand over responsibility blindly.

If you don't feel comfortable with a decision or an element of your care, it is best to get a second opinion. And even if obstetricians often meet it with derision, looking things up on the internet as a competent pregnant woman is certainly not harmful. Even doctors don't know everything. They do however sometimes worry about women showing them up by knowing more about a certain subject than them.

So, during consultations with your doctor, ask questions rather than volunteer the information gained in this way and make up your own mind from the answers.

What do your notes actually mean?

The estimated date of birth (EDB/EDD)

If you take up standard antenatal care you are generally handed a set of notes in which doctor or midwife document any examinations and test results.

When you visit your doctor or your midwife freshly pregnant, they will likely take your blood, do a risk assessment by taking your history and finally, calculate your statistically most likely EDB.

Generally, 40 weeks are added to the first day of your last period, and you end up with the 'magic date'.

At that point few pregnant women realise that this date can cause a lot of heartache later on in pregnancy as it is generally seen as risky to go over this date despite the fact that normal pregnancies statistically last around 40 weeks, +/- 2 weeks either side. This means that pregnancies lasting 38 and 42 weeks are not unusual. Even pregnancies lasting 37 weeks or 43 weeks are a normal variation of the norm. (Jukic 2013)

A birth past the estimated date of birth is perfectly normal, but once the date has passed many doctors and midwives start to become anxious – sometimes even panicky as more and more days pass.

Pressure to have increased monitoring, for example CTGs every other day and to be induced between 10-12 days over dates is common.

The reason for this is the small increase in risk for the baby from the end of the 42nd week, in the 43rd week of pregnancy and beyond. There is more in depth information about going overdue on page 82.

Your history, general test results and pregnancy specific test results

There is an official list of medical conditions and circumstances (in the German pregnancy notes, the Mutterpass, noted as catalog A and B) that make a pregnancy 'high risk'.

Risk in the medical sense does not automatically mean that there is imminent danger. Risks are determined by statistical likelihood, for example by how likely it is to suffer an adverse event with a certain condition compared to without it.

However, risk assessments like this don't necessarily apply to individual circumstances.

We could also approach it like this: The more risk factors present, the more important it is to avoid unnecessary intervention and disheartening information as well as going into an unfamiliar environment. The investigations by Marjorie Tew in the 80s very much confirm that. (Tew, 1986)

Often just one tick in a box regarding medical conditions labels you 'high risk'.

Being younger than 18 or older than 35, having birthed more than 4 children, having had complications during a previous birth can be enough.

Also on the list are history of blood clotting disorders/thromboses, allergies, obesity, skeletal/bone abnormalities, previous premature birth, previous small baby, two or more miscarriages, stillbirth, previous caesarean section or a previous pregnancy less than a year ago.

It is important to differentiate between risk factors you can prepare for and simply statistical elevations of risk.

Whether or not you are ultimately labelled as a woman with a high risk pregnancy/birth depends largely on your caregiver's assessment and perception of your risk factors.

Other reasons for a high risk label are situations that can arise during the current pregnancy: urinary tract infections, low/high blood pressure, being unsure of dates of your last period, multiple pregnancy, bleeding, premature contractions, placenta praevia, psychological/social problems, and gestational diabetes.

Again, your caregiver's assessment of any of these issues determines your individual level of risk.

The high risk label generally means closer surveillance in pregnancy, should you choose to take up the offer of maternity care. However, due to the large catalogue of conditions included in the risk assessment, nearly 70% of all pregnant women are labelled high risk in one way or another in Germany. (BQS-Bundesauswertung, 2008)

We have to wonder whether two thirds of all pregnant women really face an elevated risk as suggested in the generous application of the high risk label or if we are using that label to create more need for antenatal surveillance.

The following describes some of the tests and investigations offered under the standard model of maternity care and what their results mean. This is useful to help you decide whether you would find them helpful or would rather decline them.

Screening for sexually transmitted infections – syphilis, HIV, hepatitis B, chlamydia

This screening makes sense if you have or have had several sexual partners.

HIV and Hepatitis B should also be tested for if you have used drugs intravenously.

Screening for gestational diabetes – Glucose Tolerance Test, urinalysis

Urine is often tested for glucose when you visit your midwife or doctor. Sugar can only be present in the urine when blood sugar is also high.

A glucose tolerance test can detect a problem with your blood sugar metabolism, but not accurately.

The test is generally offered between the 24th and 28th week of pregnancy and consists of drinking 50g glucose dissolved in 200mls of liquid (this is the equivalent of approximately 33 gummy bears). Fasting is not necessary before this test, and the blood sugar is assessed an hour after the drink.

If the result is higher than 7.5mmol/l, a further test is advised. For this, the pregnant woman has to drink 300mls of water containing 75g glucose. Blood sugar is measured before drinking, as well as one hour and two hours after. The results give more in depth information about the abnormal blood sugar metabolism.

These tests may somewhat differ in the UK or other countries outside Germany, depending on area and protocol, but the gist is the same.

These glucose tolerance tests are tolerated differently by everyone. It is not rare to feel faint or sick after drinking the glucose. I know of at least one woman who reacted so violently she went into premature labour.

Some also suspect that the test can trigger gestational diabetes in itself. Therefore I feel it is overkill, counterproductive and unhealthy to test every pregnant woman in this way, as is mandatory in Austria for example.

If high blood sugars are indeed suspected, it seems more sensible and diagnostically conclusive to assess fasting levels in the morning and postprandial levels after each meal, over several days.

Additionally, pregnant women, especially those who are obese or have other risk factors for gestational diabetes, should watch their intake of carbohydrates. It is particularly important to largely avoid sugars (including hidden sugars in fruit and juice) and refined flour.

Fat does not influence blood sugar levels or tendency to put on weight, provided of course that it is not consumed to excess and only until you feel full. (Read more about fats on page 31)

Physical exercise also has a regulatory effect on blood sugar. Preventative lifestyle changes are always preferable to testing and treating with medication after the horse has already bolted.

Problems with blood sugar regulation lead to a 'high risk' label. It is often difficult to find a midwife happy to support homebirth in those circumstances. Fears mostly centre around the baby becoming too big and suffering hypoglycaemia after birth.

A prophylactic caesarean section is best declined and induction is generally not necessary either.

If blood sugar levels have been well controlled in pregnancy, either by diet or insulin, keep a positive mindset. Even big babies can be born vaginally, although on occasion it might be a slightly more difficult or longer labour.

And it is definitely worth trying to stabilise blood sugars naturally with exercise and diet.

Blood sugar can also be checked after the birth, either in the woman or, if there are any worries, the baby. Getting breastfeeding off to a good start is particularly important for diabetics and pregnant women whose levels are borderline, to avoid the baby suffering hypoglycaemia.

Rubella Titre

Rubella in pregnancy can lead to miscarriage or, if the infection occurs during embryonic/fetal organ formation in the first 12 weeks of pregnancy, it can typically lead to malformations of eyes, ears, heart and other organs. Later in pregnancy, rubella generally does not have such a drastic impact once the fetus is mostly developed and has no, or much less severe consequences.

It makes sense to check rubella antibodies if you are not sure if you have suffered rubella in the past or if your last vaccination was some time ago. It's even better to check antibodies before pregnancy though as vaccination during pregnancy is contraindicated.

It is important to be aware however that a positive antibody check does not necessarily provide 100% protection against rubella and it is possible, albeit rarely, to catch it even if vaccinated. It is also possible to have suffered from rubella (or other childhood diseases), not test positive for antibodies and still be immune.

Besides, even slapped cheek syndrome can be harmful to the newborn yet there is unfortunately no vaccination for it. In the case of rubella and slapped cheek syndrome, and many other infectious diseases, it is not only the contact with the virus that predispose infection.

The state of the mother's immune system and her nutritional status have a much bigger deciding role in contracting the disease and, in case of contracting it, its influence on the unborn.

Screening for pre-eclampsia – urinalysis, blood pressure, weight

Preeclampsia is a disorder in pregnancy that is still in part a mystery to medical science. It generally presents in the last trimester as elevated blood pressure, protein in the urine, oedema, nausea, headaches as well as fits.

Taking blood pressure, checking urine for protein and weighing the pregnant woman (which is not generally done in the UK anymore) can detect the early signs of this disorder to start treatment as soon as possible. These tests are easily done at home and all you need are scales, a blood pressure monitor and urinalysis sticks.

Preeclampsia is more common in first pregnancies, in overweight women, diabetics, twin pregnancies and women over 35. This indicates that this disorder appears when pregnancy, for whatever reasons, becomes too physically taxing.

Taking preventative measures makes sense and it is best to start prevention even before becoming pregnant by nourishing the body and giving it everything it needs to sustain a healthy pregnancy. Especially important are adequate consumption of vitamin D, protein and salt. Earlier recommendations to limit salt intake to avoid oedema possibly increase risks. Drinking the occasional glass of salt water or bone broth seasoned to taste goes a long way to covering salt and mineral intake requirements.

Haemoglobin (iron) levels

Hb stands for haemoglobin, the iron containing biomolecule that gives red blood cells their colour. Hb levels fall in every healthy pregnancy as the body carries more fluid. This is normal and should not lead to iron supplementation in itself.

As a rule, the gut increases uptake of iron from normal foods in pregnancy, but if there is cause to believe there is a genuine issue with Hb levels (pallor, excessive tiredness, pale gums, sometimes itchy skin, low iron stores detected by measuring ferritin with a blood test) assessing what may inhibit iron absorption is as important as looking at increasing iron content in food.

In any case it is recommended that the iron consumed be as bio-available as possible, which means eating iron rich foods rather than taking iron supplements. This is because iron tablets in particular can cause a problem that many pregnant women are already struggling with: constipation.

Determining your blood group and rhesus factor

Both of these are worth knowing, although many women are already aware of their blood group if they had their blood tested for other reasons or have been pregnant before. Blood group as well as rhesus factor are the expression of certain proteins on the surface of red blood cells.

If a mother is rhesus negative she does not have the rhesus factor (about 17% of the population of Central Europe doesn't). If the unborn baby does have the factor it is rhesus positive.

With this combination (mother rhesus negative, baby rhesus positive) it is possible that the mother's body may form antibodies against this rhesus factor. This can only happen if fetal blood reaches maternal circulation, either during birth or in pregnancy.

A bleed due to trauma at the placental site can cause fetal blood cells to flow into the intervillious spaces where nutrients are exchanged between womb and placenta. These bleeds are not always outwardly noticeable but can cause a feeling of localised pressure or contractions. A more common occurrence though is fetal blood mixing with the maternal blood due to premature and forceful removal of the placenta after birth.

In a subsequent pregnancy with a rhesus positive child an immune response can take place, during which those antibodies break down some of the baby's red blood cells. To prevent this (very rare) event, women are given prophylactic **anti-D injections**. These can mop up the harmful antibodies and therefore 'hide' them. Unfortunately anti-D can also cross the placenta and enter the baby's bloodstream.

It does make sense to give an anti-D injection after blunt trauma to the abdomen, after a penetrative injury to the abdomen or after caesarean section with an anterior placenta.

However, guidelines now recommend anti D prophylaxis during pregnancy, generally at around 28 weeks and after birth.

The anti-D injection contains rhesus antibodies formed by rhesus negative humans. According to the manufacturer the anti-D products (D-Gam, Partobulin, Rhophylac, Win Rho) do not contain mercury in the form of thiomersal these days. They do however contain blood products and are therefore not 100% safe with regards to blood borne diseases.

Rarely anti-D products can cause allergic reactions or fevers. One manufacturer warns of antibody elevation that could cause potentially false results during blood group and antibody tests.

Antibody titres are generally done routinely in pregnancy. This test checks if the mother's body has produced any rhesus antibodies (as well as other, less important ones).

So how do you deal with this issue as a responsible rhesus negative women?

First of all you should find out if the baby's father is rhesus positive. If he happens to be rhesus negative as well, the baby will be too and there is no need to worry about this issue anymore.

These days it is also possible to determine the fetal blood group from the 12th week of pregnancy via a blood test that analyses fetal DNA present in maternal blood.

The risk of a rhesus negative mother sensitising herself against a rhesus positive child by forming antibodies without anti-D prophylaxis is approximately 8-16% according to literature. The more traumatic the birth, the higher the risk of injury to the placental surface. A one-off injection after birth drops the risk of sensitisation to about 0.8-2% and if the antenatal prophylaxis is added, it drops again to around 0.08 or rather 0.1%.

The risk of sensitisation after miscarriage without prophylaxis is approximately 2% and rises to around 5% if a dilatation and curettage (D&C) is performed. (Cunningham 1997)

There is, however, an issue with research regarding anti-D prophylaxis. In the relevant studies, whilst blood titres were analysed, the ways in which those titres actually affected babies born to sensitised mothers were not. We don't have definitive proof that prophylaxis is effective. Equally, the studies are very small and a final assessment with regards to risks and side effects is not possible.

As seen above, maternal and fetal blood are less likely to mix in pregnancy than during birth. Many freebirthers therefore request a one-off anti D prophylaxis after birth if the baby is rhesus positive. This should happen within 72 hours after birth.

Some mothers don't have any prophylaxis if the birth was gentle and physiological and therefore low in risk with regards to a blood mixing incident – as is generally the case in freebirths. Moreover, approximately one third of mothers don't react with antibody formation, even if their blood mixes with that of their baby. (Graf 2010)

Further, sensitisation of the mother does not necessarily mean that the baby in a subsequent pregnancy will be gravely affected. Often the only thing apparent is more marked jaundice. Whether the mother's body reacts adequately to the new pregnancy or not is largely determined by the health of her immune system.

Interestingly, the baby having a blood group incompatible with the mother's provides a certain level of protection. If the fetal blood reaches the mother's circulation in this scenario it seems that the maternal antibodies quickly eliminate it and therefore only 2% as opposed to 16% become sensitised without prophylaxis. (Cunningham 1997)

Screening for chromosomal abnormalities, hereditary diseases and malformations

There are many different invasive and non-invasive tests to help detect chromosomal abnormalities and malformations in the fetus.

Ultrasound scans and a variety of blood tests to measure levels of certain hormones are generally considered non-invasive. In combination with nuchal fold measurements, they can give an indication as to the likelihood of a chromosomal abnormality.

Invasive tests, which have the potential to cause miscarriage, are amniocentesis, chorionic villi sampling and cordocentesis. Samples from these tests contain DNA of the unborn baby which can be analysed with regards to chromosomal issues.

Pregnant women after the age of 35 are often urged to accept prenatal diagnostic screening as the risk for chromosomal abnormalities, e.g. trisomy 21, increases with age. Apart from the ethical issue of eliminating certain babies as their chromosomal anomalies are considered unacceptable for parents, chromosomal testing brings up other problems too.

The whole procedure of chromosomal screening, the test itself and the waiting for results is an emotional rollercoaster ride for parents, especially the mother. Will the child be normal? How can the mother feel positive about her baby, just in case she may decide on a termination if marked chromosomal anomalies are diagnosed?

This can turn the pregnancy into a time full of worry, hope is overshadowed by fear and the mother-child bond is already conditional. For women who would never consider termination, prenatal testing may well be unnecessary.

Group B Streptococcus

Group B streptococcus (or rather beta haemolytic group B streptococcus, GBS) is a normal part of our bacterial gut flora.

Approximately 15–25% of all pregnant women are colonised with GBS in their vagina or colon. 50% of all babies born to mothers carrying these bacteria in vagina or colon pick them up during birth, but only 0.5–1% of babies go on to show subsequent signs of infection. (Katz & Moos 1994)

Preventative administration of antibiotics to the mother during birth can lower infection rates by approximately 65%. (Schrag & Zywicki 2000)

Newborn infections are no walk in the park. GBS is only one type of bacteria which can be passed from mother to baby and cause life threatening infection in some cases.

In view of this it is good to know that the bacteria in themselves are not really the bad guys occupying the vagina illegally, rather they are an indicator showing that the vaginal flora and potentially the immune system are not working optimally.

Just like nettles grow more abundantly the more nitrogen is present in the ground, GBS grows more the friendlier the vaginal flora.

Under normal circumstances this does not generally happen unless the vaginal environment is unbalanced and less acidic than normal.

Otherwise we'd have to wonder how it can be that a bacterium most people live healthy lives with can overgrow in some and cause devastating illness.

Certain bacteria and fungi love sugar. People who indulge their sweet tooth unbalance their bodies biochemically, including the bacterial flora. Urinary tract infections as well as other ascending infections in pregnancy can be a sign of this imbalance.

This is why it is advisable, as already mentioned earlier, to mostly avoid refined sugars and flour when pregnant. As a supporting measure, vaginal probiotic tablets or tampons dipped into live yogurt may be beneficial in restoring a healthy balanced vaginal flora.

Moreover, garlic is well known as an antibiotic. There are some small studies which confirm this and have found it to be effective in killing GBS (Troendle 2012). Garlic can irritate mucous membranes and should be dipped into good quality oil (e.g. olive oil) before inserting it into the vagina.

GBS colonisation status can change over a course of pregnancy, so it is possible to test positive one day and be in the clear two weeks later.

Looking at the numbers, the risk of infection is very low with GBS. Whether a newborn gets infected is not only dependent on GBS status, but also on other variables: premature birth, premature rupture of membranes or elevated temperature during birth.

Urinalysis for leukocytes and red blood cells

Urinalysis dip sticks at the midwife's or doctor's appointment can show red and white blood cells, both indicators for urinary tract infections, which are common in pregnancy. Nutritionally, the same principle as for avoiding GBS applies as mentioned earlier.

Fetal position and presentation, fundus, heartbeat and other pregnancy checks

All these things are recorded during antenatal checks:

- **What is the baby's position?**

  As soon as the baby reaches a certain size, palpation (feeling by either yourself or the midwife) or ultrasound can determine fetal position. Some of the positions determined are cephalic presentation, breech presentation, transverse lie and sometimes, when the baby is still quite small and palpation is difficult, the midwife may only be able to determine a longitudinal lie, if anything at all.

- **Where is the fundus (the top of the womb)?**

  Generally this is assessed with symphysis pubis, umbilicus and ribcage as points of reference.

  By 24 weeks of pregnancy, the fundus generally reaches the umbilicus and at the end of pregnancy it is around the same height as the ribcage but gets lower again when the head engages into the pelvis.

  Birth professionals often document fundal height by measuring the pregnant abdomen from symphysis to fundus. Each centimeter represents a week of pregnancy (see illustration).

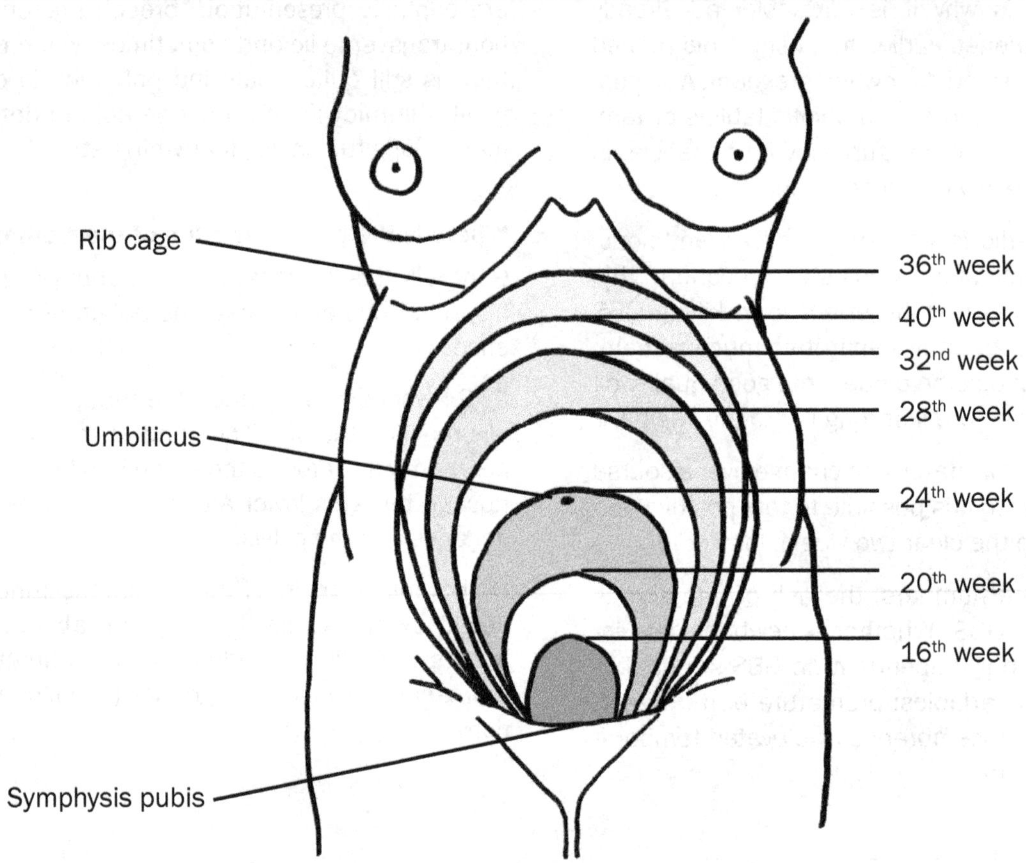
Rib cage
36th week
40th week
32nd week
28th week
Umbilicus
24th week
20th week
16th week
Symphysis pubis

Figure 1: Fundal height
Fundal height in relation to week of pregnancy

- **Is the baby's heartbeat visible or audible?**

  The fetal heartbeat can usually be detected around the 7th week of pregnancy by ultrasound or between the 10th and 14th week by doppler (Sonicaid).

  However, it is not unusual to be unable to find a heartbeat even later in pregnancy, despite the heart beating away without problems. This can greatly unsettle a pregnant woman and listening in later rather than earlier may be a good idea.

  As soon as movements from the baby can be felt, listening in to the heartbeat becomes unnecessary, at least for the mother. After all, where there is movement there is a heartbeat.

- **Is there any swelling or varicose veins?**
- **How much does the pregnant woman weigh?**
- **What is the blood pressure?**
- **Were any issues detected during urinalysis?**
- **What were the findings from any vaginal examinations?**
- **HB levels** (if bloods were taken)
- **Any other relevant results.**

Ultrasound

Ultrasound was 'invented' in the Second World War to help detect enemy submarines. Soon its potential for medical purposes was discovered.

Ultrasound utilises sound waves at a frequency not audible to the human ear to produce images of bodily structures and tissues. Depending on density, tissues and fluids reflect those sound waves at varying strengths. Computers can transform this feedback into accurate, sometimes even three dimensional pictures.

During the 1970s, doctors started to use ultrasound to find answers to questions arising during high risk pregnancies. Quite some time has passed since then and ultrasound is now routine for almost all pregnancies and births.

Germany was the first country to start using ultrasound routinely and still remains the country with most frequent use of this technology. (Erikson 2008)

If the use of ultrasound had made pregnancy safer, it would perhaps be possible to ignore the fact that it has never been appropriately researched with regards to its potential effects on the unborn baby. The fact that false positives during ultrasound examinations contribute to the boom in caesarean sections whilst overall safety remains unchanged for mother and baby (Ewigman 1993) leads to the interpretation that routine ultrasound may be detrimental to the health of mother and baby.

Various studies not only point towards a potential to damage the DNA, cells and in particular the brain, but have also found a higher risk for heart defects, language delay and behavioural issues as well as miscarriage, prematurity and stillbirth. (Lorenz 1990, Saari-Kemppainen 1990, Davies 1992, Newnham 1993, Cambell 1993, Beech 1996, Ang 2006)

Many experts are particularly critical about doppler scans to measure blood flow through maternal and fetal blood vessels (Davies 1992) as well as early pregnancy scans up to the 12th week of pregnancy when organ formation is still taking place (Chervenak 1999). Moreover, direct scans of the fetal skull are suspected to have a negative influence on brain development (Tarantal 1993, Ang 2006).

There are also some studies that did not find a connection between ultrasound examination and fetal development. (Torloni 2009)

However, the studies mentioned are mostly from the beginning of the 1990s or older. Ultrasound intensity has increased six to eight fold since then, so the subject of routine ultrasound remains controversial and the question of safety has not yet been fully answered. This is why many experts recommend women only have the bare minimum number of scans to avoid unnecessary exposure. (Caviness & Grant 2006)

Many pregnant women await their scans in feverish anticipation and fear and are very relieved when they get the confirmation all is well afterwards. In the first trimester of pregnancy it is possible to trust our instincts but it really is difficult to find anything else to reassure us, due to not yet being able to feel the baby.

Only ultrasound can actually show us what is happening inside of us. But is it sensible, just because it is possible?

Besides the potential effects on the newborn, sonographers can get it wrong in their pursuit to assess the health of the baby. I have read many an account where a baby was presumed dead (a heartbeat could not be detected repeatedly and a D&C was recommended) but turned out to be alive after all and developed normally.

It might not be a frequent occurrence but presumably pregnancies that were perfectly normal and wished for, have ended in scenarios such as this.

These scan results don't save lives, but satisfy curiosity and reduce fear temporarily. The uterus expels the embryo sooner or later and induces a miscarriage, should it really be dead. If it is alive, it will continue to develop.

Generally it does not cause a problem to carry an embryo that has passed away for a few days or weeks. Normally our bodies are very efficient at initiating miscarriage, and if the mother wants to await events naturally, a D&C or induction is not necessary. Rarely it may become necessary to seek medical attention in the case of fever or prolonged bleeding.

When it comes to detecting abnormalities at a later stage of pregnancy, ultrasound can be justified for many. Some women feel intuitively that their baby is somehow different, but some do not. Many women consciously decide on an ultrasound around the 20th week of pregnancy to exclude major abnormalities and to determine placental location.

It is pertinent to remember that ultrasound scans are not a 100% reliable diagnosis when it comes to malformations. Often anomalies are found that are not actually present and, vice versa, actual issues (sometimes major ones) are overlooked. (Chan 1997, Ewigman 1993)

Another issue relates to growth scans. Babies can be suddenly found to be too small or too large, head circumferences too small or too large. Often caesarean sections are recommended as big babies are obviously difficult to birth and the small ones need to be delivered to protect them from harm in utero.

All the while it is well known that weight calculations from scan and mathematical formulas using scan measurements have an average deviation of 350–500 grams from the actual weight of the baby. (Frimmel 2004)

Ultrasound can provide countless reasons as to why a pregnancy should not be left to run its natural course. In reality, particularly the growth assessment via scan is a very inaccurate science, probably too inaccurate to have drastic consequences such as major abdominal surgery.

An experienced midwife is often more adept at estimating the baby's weight by feeling the abdomen with her hands so there is no need to be pushed into intervention by a set of computer calculations.

I worried for a long time during my first pregnancy because a scan had detected a moderate degree of hydronephrosis (renal pelvic dilatation) in my baby. It was recommended that I have amniocentesis to rule out the chromosomal abnormality trisomy 21, despite the fact that the link between hydronephrosis and this chromosomal issue is so tenuous that most experts only urge amniocentesis if other issues are apparent. (Corteville 1992)

I declined the test due to the risk of potentially losing a healthy child during this intervention. And I would not have terminated a disabled baby anyway.

I was checked over again and again in the following weeks and the hydronephrosis reduced more and more as the baby grew bigger. Still, the worries took away a lot of joy in my pregnancy, completely unnecessarily as it turned out. My baby was born in perfect health.

This is why I decided to deal only with normal pregnancy fears as and when they happen and decline scans in future pregnancies.

Those who don't want to expose their babies to ultrasound waves also need to know that the doppler (Sonicaid) midwives use to listen to the babies heart beat, CTG machines and even devices such as Angelsounds for use by parents at home use the same technology.

You can ask your midwife to use a Pinard, if she wants to listen to the baby. This is made from wood and free from ultrasound. The Pinard can even be used by fathers and siblings to listen to the baby's heart with a little bit of practice. A normal stethoscope does not normally work, but a fetoscope is useful too. This is a device, much like a stethoscope, but better at channeling the fetal heart tones acoustically.

And even simpler: the father-to-be can listen to his baby by putting his ear directly on his partner's belly.

Possible models of care

Depending on preference and situation, every pregnant woman can decide for herself who she would like to provide her care during pregnancy, birth and the postnatal period – or not, as the case may be.

Following are some possible models of care:

- Antenatal care with midwife or doctor, birth at the hospital, postnatal care at home with the midwife. This is the classic and most common model of care.

- Antenatal care, home or birth centre birth and postnatal care at home with a midwife. You can keep open the option of freebirth by calling the midwife later or when needed.

- Antenatal and postnatal care with midwife, self-directed birth.

- Self-directed pregnancy and birth, postnatal care by midwife. If the woman already has several children, she may appreciate the attention and a listening ear.

- Self-directed pregnancy, birth and postnatal period, supported by other women on the internet and/or real life, the partner, a midwife at the end of a phone etc.

Common pregnancy ailments

The following tips and tricks are not necessarily universally known, but can be very helpful:

Nausea

Women who suffer from this have a hard time, without a doubt. To a certain degree, nausea can be considered a normal phenomenon which normally disappears sometime before the 20th week of pregnancy.

However, it has been observed that pregnancy nausea is unknown in many non-Western societies. Severe pregnancy nausea is linked to low levels of magnesium, vitamin B6, folic acid and zinc.

Improving intake of those vitamins and minerals is certainly recommended and if nutrition has been below par for some time, it is worth improving stores even before pregnancy.

If nausea persists, here are some home remedies and tips:

- **Eat something** before getting up, and eat smaller meals throughout the day. You are more likely to feel sick on an empty stomach. When I was feeling sick at the beginning of my pregnancies I was constantly eating something. See what works for you. Sweets and fast food are still not recommended.

- If you can't even keep down liquids, suck on **ice cubes** or put a slice of lemon into your water. The smell of lemon soothes the stomach.

- Eat foods **rich in vitamin B6**! You can find some examples on page 35. The American College of Obstetricians and Gynaecologists (ACOG) recommends vitamin B6 as the first port of call when suffering pregnancy sickness. If it is possible, raise level with diet but it is also possible to use supplements.

- Eat foods **rich in magnesium**! Some examples on page 34.

- If you are vomiting a lot, be mindful not only of the potential for dehydration but also of the loss of **salts and minerals**. Homemade bone broth is ideal to counteract this.

- Drink **ginger tea** or take a ginger supplement. Studies have found ginger to reduce episodes of sickness and vomiting more effectively than a placebo after 6–9 days and is similar in effectiveness to vitamin B6. (Matthews 2010)

- Try **diffusing essential oils**.

Sciatica

Approximately 30 years ago, Helmut Aigelsreiter, expert in movement and training education from the Bundesanstalt für Leibeserziehung (National Institute for Physical Education) in Graz, found that most cases of sciatica were due to a shortening of a certain muscle, the piriformis.

This deep seated gluteal muscle is responsible for lateral rotation of the femur and hip extension. It needs plenty of room to effectively work for hip extension. If this muscle is shortened it presses on the sciatic nerve during extension and causes the typical sciatica pain, mostly when standing.

Stretching the affected muscles can relieve sciatic pain, even in pregnancy. Special mobility work as recommended by Aigelsreiter can be effective: Lie on your back or sit up, bend the leg on the side you want to stretch and let it drop to the side, then move your foot over the bent knee of the opposite side. Now grab the knee on the side you are aiming to stretch and pull it gently towards your chest. Hold this position for at least 30 seconds and relax into the strong stretching sensation you are likely to feel. Aim to keep your bottom on the floor or chair.

It is important to repeat this exercise several times a day and soon some relief should come, if not complete relief (Aigelsreiter 2012).

Varicose veins

Here I will tell you a story to illustrate how fear can attract the exact thing you are trying to avoid.

My mother suffered from spider and varicose veins after her 5 children were born. I assumed I would have inherited the tendency towards that affliction and was convinced the same fate would befall me if I didn't take preventative measures. I had a special pair of compression tights made in my first pregnancy.

Until then I never suffered from varicose veins before but because I was spending a lot of time standing up in operating theatres in my training, surely it would be a good idea – or so I thought. However this specially made garment creased terribly at the back of my knees when I sat down, but of course I wore it again in my second pregnancy as I was still working in hospitals for a while and stood in the operating theatres. But this time the creases behind my knees caused me phlebitis. I stopped wearing the tights but it was too late.

The phlebitis healed fully but left me with a varicose vein that is very noticeable and bothersome when I have my period or am pregnant. Now I really DO need compression tights in pregnancy. Without them the varicose vein I caused myself hurts.

Now I only wear below the knee support stockings. They do the job without squishing the back of my knee or other delicate spots.

Women who don't have any issues do not need compression garments in pregnancy. Support stockings can however be helpful if you are required to sit or stand for long periods at a time, perhaps for work or during air travel. I would always prefer stockings as opposed to tights due to the problems mentioned above.

To avoid varicosities, keep mobile, put your legs up now and then and keep circulation going by pulling your toes up, holding and relaxing again. It is also important to pay attention to diet as it is not only genes that determine the elasticity of the connective tissues but also nutrient and vitamin intake.

And if those dreaded veins do appear, don't fear. Most pregnancy induced varicose veins disappear again after the birth. If not, carry them with dignity as a memento of those 9 magical months.

The symphysis and other joints

Pregnancy hormones cause many different changes in the female body. One of the changes is the loosening of the pelvic joints and ligaments to prepare the body for birth and to make room for the baby to be born.

Most women don't notice any drastic changes but towards the end of pregnancy, some women can't move without pain.

I personally didn't have problems with any joints in my first pregnancy. But particularly in the third and fourth I noticed stabbing pains in the symphysis pubis and in the sacroiliac joint (where sacrum and ilium meet) at certain times.

Particularly during my third pregnancy, the pain started so early that at times I wondered how I would manage the rest of the pregnancy, if I was already in so much pain when moving around now?

I researched my problem and from then on tried to mostly move symmetrically so that the joint surfaces would move against each other as little as possible and therefore not cause me too much pain. Getting out of bed, gently and with knees together, avoiding asymmetrical weight distribution with relation to my hips and standing in a symmetrical fashion all helped.

After I had swapped all painful movements for pain free ones for a few days, the overall pain lessened and eventually almost completely disappeared. In my fourth pregnancy I already knew what I had to do when the twinges started again.

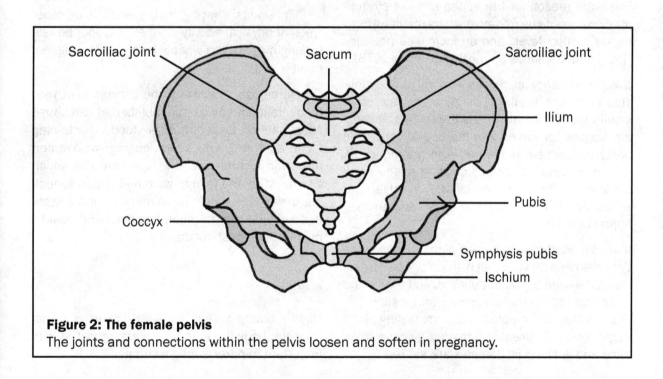

Figure 2: The female pelvis
The joints and connections within the pelvis loosen and soften in pregnancy.

Stretch marks

You can avoid stretch marks if you keep applying creams to your bump and do a sort of plucking massage. Sounds familiar? It seems this is not actually true at all. All the creams and massages in the world do not seem to influence stretch mark formation at all, at least this is what the evidence says. (Young 2012)

Interestingly, not every woman gets stretch marks. Do some women have stronger connective tissues than others?

Getting stretch marks is more likely under the following conditions: obesity, excessive weight gain in pregnancy, alcohol consumption and having a larger than average baby. (Osman 2007, J-Orh 2008)

Intriguingly, stretch marks also often appear on people taking the medication cortisone or who have a condition where their bodies produce too much cortisol (the body's very own version of cortisone). Diabetes and puberty also result in stretchmarks for some people.

The main reason for the appearance of stretchmarks seems to be oxidative stress resulting from higher cortisol levels and an increased need for zinc due to demands on the body (Huber 1978).

Every pregnancy increases cortisol production. This increases insulin resistance and therefore insulin production also rises to rapidly transport any sugars consumed into the body's cells. This basic mechanism is the same in pregnancy as it is in all other conditions causing raised cortisol levels. With good nutrition, low in sugar and a healthy lifestyle the female body can generally adjust beautifully.

If insulin production has been high for quite some time, perhaps due to a diet high in sugars, cortisol levels may already be out of sync. Add to that the hormonal changes in pregnancy and insulin production may not be able to keep up, raising blood sugar levels. Noticeably impaired glucose tolerance and gestational diabetes are the result.

Cortisol levels are raised in every pregnancy, but only occasionally do they reach such a level that the whole system is thrown off balance. And if the metabolism has to function under stress, zinc will also be used at higher levels. Zinc stores are low in humans generally and deficiency often results in stretchmarks. (Watts 1988, Nriagu 2007, Stamm 2009)

However it is not known whether it is the stress on the metabolism and the associated decreased zinc levels or the elevated cortisol or perhaps the combination of both that cause the stretchmarks. Other metabolic factors may also play a role.

Constipation

Anything that gives you a deep feeling of relaxation is also likely to give your gut motility a boost. Finding out what gives you that feeling of relaxation and the ability to open your bowels may also make clear which conditions are going to be most helpful for you when giving birth.

It might be a walk in the woods, a look at your book case, a little bit of unselfconscious dancing in the kitchen or other types of physical activity ... What gets your bowels moving may also be what is helpful in the big moment.

Of course you should also be conscious of your fluid intake and avoid iron tablets that can cause constipation. Sauerkraut or foods containing lactic acid can help keep you regular. Women are often recommended a high fibre diet which can backfire and lead to wind and generally feeling unwell. So simply avoiding cake and sweets and keeping your nutrition balanced and healthy might be the best option.

Muscle cramps

Nightly cramp should be regarded as a signal from the body to fill up its mineral stores. A very important mineral is magnesium.

When I suffered nightly calf cramps again and again, just one tablet of magnesium seemed to do the trick.

Generally food sources are preferable to supplements. With supplements comes the risk of overdose which can lead to a drop in blood pressure or the inability of the uterus to produce strong contractions due to its action as a muscle relaxant.

More information about appropriate foods can be found on page 29. Magnesium is not always effective and it is always pertinent to investigate for deficiencies in other minerals.

Dental caries

Other causes for caries besides sugar intake include lack of fat-soluble vitamins in the diet and the increased need for calcium in pregnancy and breastfeeding.

2 teaspoons of fermented cod liver oil with its high amount of fat-soluble vitamins help remineralise teeth and can halt caries in its tracks. More about this in the book 'Cure Tooth Decay'. (Nagel 2011)

Self-directed Pregnancy

You are free to create your own antenatal care if you decide to opt out of the standard system of care provision.

You can find out more about you and your baby than you think, even without medical gadgets and tests. If you want to take up any tests or examinations as listed in 'What do your notes actually mean' (page 43) you can get a doctor or in most cases a midwife to do them for you.

If you have already had a baby and you have already had some of the tests or they just don't seem sensible to you, you are free to go without.

Your baby will grow regardless and you can answer many questions yourself with plenty of background knowledge and sensible awareness.

What position is the baby in?

While preparing for birth it makes sense to determine the baby's position.

If the baby is already in a good longitudinal position, it is reasonable to assume the birth will be quick and uncomplicated. If the baby is not in an optimal position you can take measures to change its position into a more advantageous one.

Figuring out where the baby is lying is not normally particularly difficult in the last two months of pregnancy. The closer the birth, the stronger the baby and it's kicks and movements.

If you want to find out which way the baby is lying, you do it by feeling your belly, just like the midwife would. For this, you lie down on your back, with your knees bent, relax your abdominal muscles and feel your belly with both hands – from left side to the middle, from the right to the middle and from the top of the uterus downwards.

Even earlier in pregnancy you can monitor the baby's growth and the progress of pregnancy by checking the fundal height – how far the top of the uterus has risen out of the pelvis (see illustration on page 50).

The fundus is at its highest around the 36th week of pregnancy, right under the ribcage and then lowers down again as the pregnancy progresses due to the head engaging in the pelvis and the uterus positioning itself 'in line' with the birth canal. The head generally engages earlier in first time mothers than in mothers who have already birthed a baby.

It is not uncommon for second or subsequent babies to only engage in the pelvis just before birth or indeed during birth.

Sometimes, towards the end of pregnancy, the baby kicking or you giving your uterus a good poke can set off a Braxton Hicks (practice) contraction, which makes your whole belly go hard. Of course you can't feel a thing then apart from the powerful strong muscle that is your uterus.

But when your belly has relaxed again, you can often feel something long and solid on one side. This is your baby's **back**. The other side is usually soft.

If the baby is **head down** as they usually are, you can feel the head over your symphysis pubis. If the head is already engaged in the pelvis you can feel it internally through your vagina. This is usually easiest with an empty bladder, in a half squat with your index and middle finger.

The baby's **feet** make themselves felt by strong kicks on the opposite side of the baby's back. The baby's bottom is the extension of its back and generally feels like a round firm dome.

The baby's **hands** feel like little butterfly wings at the bottom of your bump, just over your symphysis either on the left or right. Later, when fingernails have grown, you can sometimes feel the baby's hands as an unpleasant scratching sensation.

The cephalic presentation (that means the baby is **head down**) with the baby's back on the right or left side is the most common position a baby takes up for birth.

It is also called **occipitoanterior position**, because the baby's occiput (the back of the head) is in the anterior (frontal) portion of the pelvis. This is a good starting position and most babies are born that way.

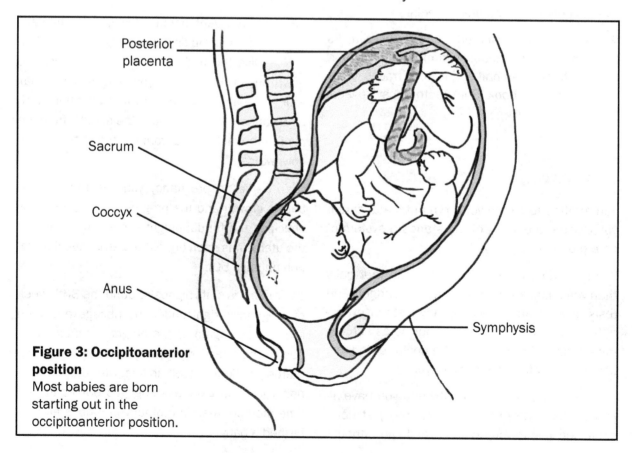

Figure 3: Occipitoanterior position
Most babies are born starting out in the occipitoanterior position.

Another variation of the occipitoanterior position is the baby with its back directly in the middle of the mother's bump. With the mother on all fours, the baby is almost nestled in the mother's abdomen like in a hammock. Kicks can hardly be felt as they are directed towards the mother's spine. Mothers with a baby in this position have often already had more than one baby, and there is a little more room in their uterus. These babies are also born easily.

A little less ideal as a starting point is the **occipito-posterior position**. In this position, the back of the baby's head is directed towards the posterior (rear) portion of the pelvis, its back towards your back. Tummy and legs are towards the mother's abdominal wall and kicks are predominantly felt towards the front. A baby in this position will be born with its face towards the mothers front, unless it turns during birth. When the head is born, it will face the same direction as you.

A baby born like this is called a '**stargazer**'. This term has likely been coined in recent times in which women usually birthed their babies either lying down or in the semirecumbent position. When the head is born, the baby 'gazes at the stars', so to say.

During an occipitoposterior birth, the head can't tuck in optimally to enter the pelvis with the smallest possible diameter, and therefore these labours are often more protracted and difficult, typically with backache. Many women have had their home-birth dreams shattered by this. It makes sense to encourage the baby into a more advantageous starting position with the following advice about posture.

It is speculated that the increase in occipitoanterior births is due to us spending more time reclined comfortably in front of the TV, or hunched up in front of a computer. We rarely squat or go on all fours, to scrub floors for example. The fact that birth commonly takes place in the semirecumbent position is also thought to contribute to this increase.

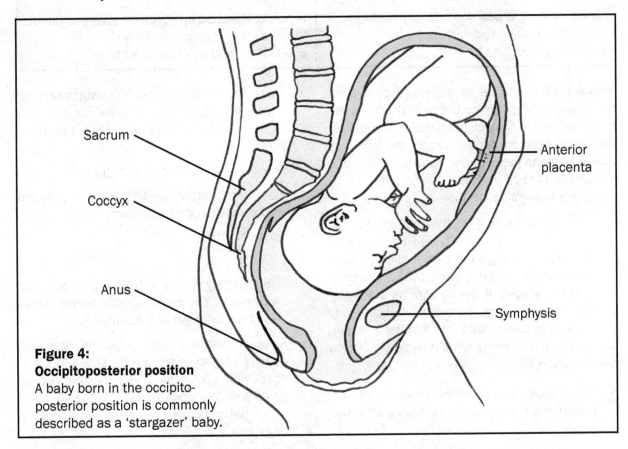

Figure 4:
Occipitoposterior position
A baby born in the occipito-posterior position is commonly described as a 'stargazer' baby.

Sacrum

Coccyx

Anus

Anterior placenta

Symphysis

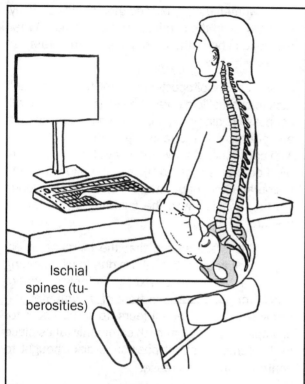

Figure 5: Upright position + fetal positioning
An upright position encourages a
optimal fetal position for birth.

Ischial
spines (tu-
berosities)

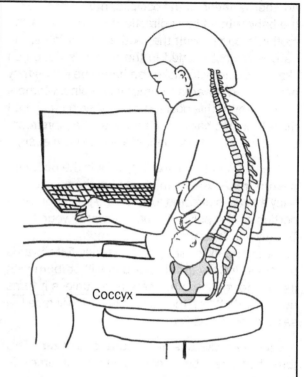

Figure 6: Hunched up posture + fetal positioning
Hunched up posture can lead to
suboptimal fetal positioning for birth.

Coccyx

Sloppy posture (Figure 6) is marked by a tilted pelvis and sitting on your coccyx, instead of distributing your body's weight on the ischial spines. As can be seen on the illustration, the coccyx is pushed into the pelvis during hunched sitting and the back has to compensate for the pelvic tilt by being in a hunchback position.

Frequent sitting like this (not only in front of the computer, but also on the sofa), can encourage the baby's back to lie in the curve of the maternal back. Unless the baby turns at some point, it will be born as a stargazer. This can make birth more difficult, as already mentioned. To coax a baby into a better position, you can do the following while pregnant (El Harta 1995, Sutton 1996):

- Spend some time on all fours daily, especially when the baby appears to be having an active phase.

- Three times daily, spend 20 minutes on your knees, with your bottom in the air and your chest close to the floor (Knee-chest-position, Figure 8b)

- Make sure you sit with a straight back

- Either kneel or sit upright, perhaps propped with a V-pillow or on a kneeling chair.

- Go swimming

- Do Yoga

- Dance or stay mobile with other gentle, varied movements. The baby learns movement patterns from the mother's activity.

- Squat: regularly practice squatting down. It doesn't have to be a deep squat, a supported squat with a low stool under your bottom will do as well (but don't hunch your back). More about pelvic floor exercise and squatting on page 132.

Breech presentation

A baby that is lying with its bottom down in the pelvis can be detected by feeling its head directly under the mother's ribs. It is much more firm than a baby's bottom and one mother told me that she can tell it is the head by getting it to tuck in when poking it. This is most definitely not possible with the baby's bottom. If the bottom is down in the pelvis, it is also possible to feel kicks into your bladder.

More about birth with a breech baby on page 106.

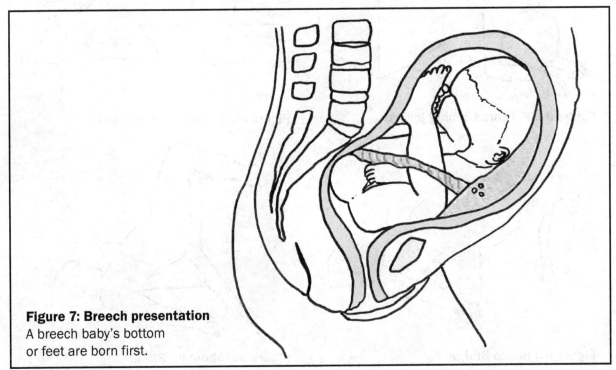

Figure 7: Breech presentation
A breech baby's bottom
or feet are born first.

The following exercises can help turn a baby from a breech to a cephalic presentation (Tully 2012). Illustration on next page.

> Please make sure you tolerate these exercises and don't feel unwell during them. If you feel unwell or sick, the baby may mirror this, so it would be better to try other alternatives.

- Kneel on the sofa and put your hands on the floor, for approximately 30 seconds, two or three times daily (forward leaning inversion, Figure 8a)
- Spend time in an all fours position, especially when the baby is active
- Lying on the floor, rest your legs on the sofa and elevate your hips with a pillow or similar, once or twice a day, for about 10–15 minutes (Indian Bridge, Figure 8c)
- Head or shoulder stand (Figure 8d)
- Lean a board (for example an ironing board) against the sofa and stop slippage with cushions or similar, then lie down on the board, with your head on the low end, for 20 minutes, three times daily (breech tilt, Figure 8e)
- Lie on your side, close to the edge of the sofa (get someone to support you so you don't fall) and let your upper leg drop down the edge of the sofa without twisting your hips or the rest of your body. This exercise is called 'side-lying release' and is supposed to release muscles in the pelvis to enable the baby to engage its head (Figure 8f).

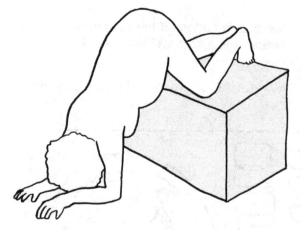

Figure 8a: Forward Leaning Inversion

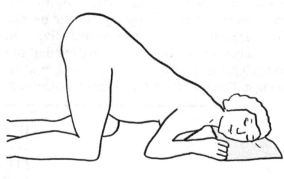

Figure 8b: Knee-Chest-Position

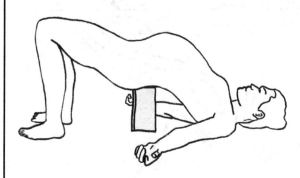

Figure 8c: Indian Bridge

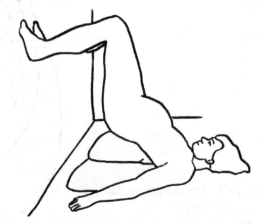

Figure 8d: Shoulder Stand

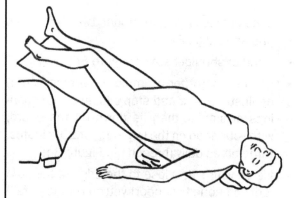

Figure 8e: Breech Tilt

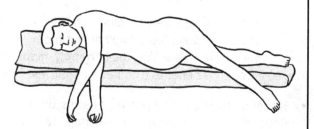

Figure 8f: Side-Lying Release

Figure 8a–8f: Exercises for optimal fetal positioning
Different exercises can help to optimise the baby's position before or during birth.

Transverse and oblique lie

In the weeks before birth, babies are rarely in a **transverse or oblique lie**.

The **transverse lie** is hard to miss. Unlike a breech presentation, a transverse lie is impossible to birth naturally. The baby's spine forming a cross with yours, you can feel the bottom on one side (right or left) and the head on the opposite. The back is lying across your belly and your belly bulges on both sides.

An **oblique lie** is not quite so easy to detect. The head is not central in the pelvis but sits just off centre over the top of the pelvis.

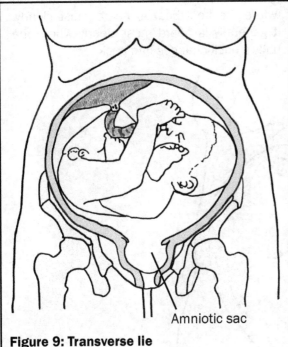

Amniotic sac

Figure 9: Transverse lie
The spine of a baby in transverse lie forms a cross with the mother's spine.

Transverse and oblique lies can occur when there is a lot of amniotic fluid (polyhydramnios), fibroids (benign growths in the uterus) are present, a placenta is in the way or the mother has simply had several babies before and there is plenty of room. It could also be the case that the natural inclination to be head down is not present in the baby just yet.

Most babies however do turn head down eventually if we give them time, either before birth or when contractions have started. The same exercises as for breech babies can be used to coax a transverse or oblique baby into the pelvis.

Whenever a baby is reluctant to engage into the pelvis, treatment by an osteopath, chiropractor or another manual therapist can be helpful. Adjusting and aligning the pelvis can make it easier for the baby to find the optimal position for birth.

You can also talk to your baby if it is in a suboptimal position for birth. Even though of course they won't understand word for word, they can feel your intention in a certain way and often respond with swift turning manoeuvers. It can be particularly helpful to clearly imagine for yourself, where exactly you want your baby to be and support the move with your own hands. It seems some children already require firm guidance at a very young age.

Other ways to determine the baby's position

If you have a **fetoscope** – a device similar to a stethoscope to listen to the baby's heartbeat – you can use the location in which you can hear the heartbeat the clearest to determine the baby's position. Or you can ask someone to find the heartbeat with a **Pinard**.

Personally, I didn't find a **stethoscope** helpful in finding the fetal heartbeat. Apart from some exceptions I mostly found my uterine artery pulse and the whooshing of the placental vessels, despite trying hard. In any case, if using one, don't touch the tubes of the stethoscope while listening in and use the bell rather than the membrane to listen if possible.

Another indicator of baby's position is where you can feel **hiccups**, because the origin of the hiccups is the diaphragm. Right up until the end of pregnancy there is nothing so noticeable, apart from movements, as the baby's recurring, sometimes violent, hiccups. This strengthens the diaphragmatic muscles used by the baby to inflate its lungs and breathe after birth.

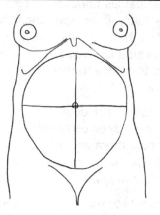

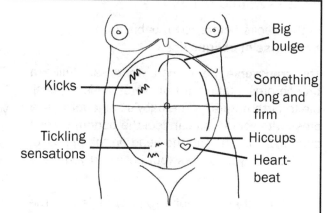

Figure 10a: Belly map for movements
Create a map to track movement: draw your belly as a circle, your belly button is the centre. Divide the circle into 4 parts as shown.

Figure 10b: Mark down movement
Mark, where you can feel movement, where you can feel different parts of the baby and where the heartbeat is heard most clearly. It generally is heard most clearly where the baby's back changes into neck.

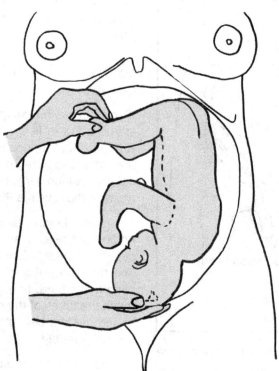

Figure 10c: Doll as a prop
With a jointed doll and your drawn up map as a guide you will now be able to mimic your baby's position. Most often the baby's back is on the left side of the uterus. This is why these illustrations show the baby's back on the left too. All these positions can of course also have the back on the right side.

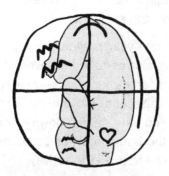 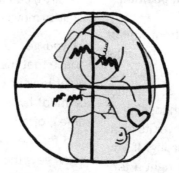 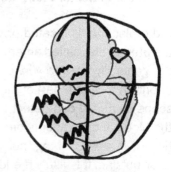

Figure 10d: Belly map with occipitoanterior position

Figure 10e: Belly map with occipitoposterior position

Figure 10f: Belly map with breech presentation

Figure 10a–10f: Instructions to determine the baby's position
Simple measures can help you find your baby's position yourself.

Where is the placenta?

Asking about the position of the placenta is helpful in determining the presence or absence of a **placenta praevia**.

A placenta praevia covers the cervical opening (os) either partially or fully, a rare but potentially dangerous situation for mother and baby. If the cervix starts opening, the placenta can shear off the uterine wall, cause haemorrhage and compromise the baby's blood supply.

A placenta that covers the os fully around the time of birth is unfortunately a definite indication for a caesarean section. At the latest it will make itself known with the start of contractions which will cause more blood loss than normal, but usually it becomes apparent much earlier in pregnancy.

I have heard old reports of old school rural midwives managing to deliver baby and placenta rapidly, saving mother and baby, but I would not recommend trying that out in this day and age and with all the medical help available nowadays. Such a case is very rare anyway.

More common is a low lying placenta that encroaches on the cervical opening. Those cases are generally diagnosed in the first or second trimester. Recurring bleeds are a typical symptom in the second trimester in particular.

The growth of the lower uterine segment (or the uterine isthmus, that is inbuilt as safety for an incidence such as this, and stretches from approximately 5mm to 4cm) lets the placenta 'migrate' upwards throughout the pregnancy and in most cases away from the cervix.

For someone with a previous caesarean section it might be worth checking placental location as it can implant into the scar and cause issues with placental separation after birth. This can, of course, only happen with an anterior placenta. The most accurate method to determine placental position is an ultrasound scan. It is also possible to determine placental position by listening for the typical 'whooshing' sounds it makes with a stethoscope (as long as it is on the front wall of the uterus).

An experienced midwife may also be able to help and feel for it by its more 'doughy' texture.

The baby's movement can also give clues. Most babies face their placenta. This is logical as the umbilical cord is connected to the middle of the placenta. It is also why babies are more frequently oblique or transverse if the placenta is low lying.

Here a list of indicators for placental position:

- If the placenta is located on the front wall of the uterus, also called anterior placenta, kicks are generally felt in a very cushioned fashion or only in a certain part of the bump. A stethoscope or pinard can detect the whooshing of the blood in the placenta directly over its location (It is a whooshing, not a pulsing. If you hear pulsing, it is likely the left or right artery supplying the uterus with blood.) The baby's heartbeat can often be heard on the side of your belly.

- If the placenta is close to or in front of the cervical opening (placenta praevia marginalis, also low lying placenta or placenta praevia totalis) you will likely experience recurring 'warning' bleeds in pregnancy or a bigger bleed at the onset of contractions.

- Concluding from all the above, it is likely to be a posterior placenta (placenta on the back wall of the uterus) if you can't hear anything on the front side of your uterus, you can feel kicks clearly all over and you don't have any bleeds. A placenta on the posterior wall of the uterus can't implant itself into a previous caesarean section scar as that is always on the anterior side of the uterus.

Is the baby well?

Once the uncertain early pregnancy phase is over, the mother will soon feel the gentle, long awaited fluttering in her belly. A sensation that gets stronger every day and with which the baby communicates: 'Hi mum, here I am. I'm alive and growing!'

Until and even during birth, the baby's movements are the most important indicator of its well being and even more meaningful than listening to the baby's heartbeat. A baby that is at risk (either in pregnancy or during birth) can maintain a 'normal' heart rate but is likely to move less or stop altogether.

As you get further into your pregnancy, you will notice that there are also certain times when it is quiet in your belly. That's when the baby sleeps, calmed by your steps and movement. Other times, often when you have settled down in your bed for the night, the baby becomes active and often gets the hiccups from all the activity.

Mostly quiet times change into times where it seems like your womb dweller is changing the wallpaper and rearranging the furniture in your belly. Even now, your baby has phases of active development and quiet, relaxed phases, just like it will have when born.

Freebirth for a first baby?

Only very few first babies are born in their own four walls, and planned freebirths in this situation are extremely rare.

There are several reasons: a woman lacks experience with a first baby, she is not sure what birth feels like and what she is likely to need. Because of that, she often doesn't have the courage and confidence to follow her gut and do what she secretly really wants for her birth. She comes to the obvious conclusion to trust the ones who are officially considered to be the experts when it comes to birth, 'just in case'.

Generally this expert ends up being a midwife or doctor for antenatal care and a hospital for birth, preferably with a newborn intensive care unit, seeing as (nearly) all women seem to choose this. A pregnancy makes you adaptable to a new baby, but also to societal norms.

The first birth experience often changes things though and more second and subsequent babies are born in birthing centres or at home.

Most first time mums who choose a homebirth have a midwife in attendance.

The birth of a first baby usually lasts longer than the birth of subsequent children. This might be because a first time mum tends to interpret any twinges as the start of labour while women with other children are more likely to ignore the sensations as long as possible and keep themselves occupied. If the first birth is a planned homebirth it is more likely to end with a hospital transfer than the birth of later siblings. (Brocklehurst 2011)

It certainly seems like a first baby needs to work hard to be born while the way for siblings appears 'paved' already. For a first birth, patience and confidence are incredibly important and you are more likely to have those in your own home than in the hospital. Optimally, one would have an experienced, calm midwife to call when needed and who'd only suggest transfer when really necessary. But if your confidence in birth is already irrefutable with your first baby, all the better.

Is it twins?

This is a question that will often come up for women who have a self-directed pregnancy. Clear indications for a twin pregnancy are:

- two heartbeats can be heard at the same time or in two different places

- the fundus (top of the uterus) grows faster than during a previous singleton pregnancy or the fundus is taller than it should be for the week of pregnancy you are in.

- lots of movement in lots of different places

- two big parts can be felt at the same time (such as 2 heads)

- women often have a dream about twin pregnancy

Being pregnant with twins means taking extra good care of yourself and your nutrition, so that your body can manage the strain of growing 2 babies until the end. This much is true for singleton and twin pregnancies: The healthier and more robust the mother and the better her nutrition and exercise during pregnancy, the lower the chance of complications.

I can also understand that a woman might not want to know that she is pregnant with twins. The pressure to accept lots of tests and monitoring, having a hospital birth in the name of safety with doctors and possibly a planned caesarean section is hard to ignore. The already booked homebirth midwife may not be willing to lend support anymore and not only does the chance of a dream birth disappear, she also has to prepare for a no doubt very turbulent first year after the birth.

Before the era of ultrasounds, surprise twin births were not uncommon. What a surprise to find 2 babies! What a shock. Much worry was avoided that way. I can certainly understand how the 'right not to know' exists in medicine.

However, being aware of what may await you allows appropriate planning or indeed a changing of plans – which is good practice for life with small children! For me personally, it would for example be important to have another helping hand present, ideally a calm, experienced midwife. It can certainly happen that the second twin needs to be born quickly or has some trouble transitioning into extrauterine life. I would not want to be alone in that case.

Studies seem to suggest that twin pregnancies are associated with a higher risk of complications, but many of those risks can be minimised with sensible nutrition and lifestyle.

This is why I would like to encourage every single woman to walk her path with determination and, after informing herself extensively, choose what is right for her in her particular set of circumstances.

Unfortunately fewer and fewer twins are born naturally due to safety concerns these days. This is why it is especially difficult to achieve a birth free of intervention in a clinical setting with twins on board.

For this reason alone, I would prefer a birth at home to a hospital one, even for two babies, as long as the pregnancy was normal.

Unfortunately, the knowledge about the different sort of safety that comes with a birth in private is scarce, so that pregnant women who are not experienced doctors or midwives themselves, easily find themselves having a wobble during their decision making.

Bleeding

Bleeds can have a variety of reasons. In early pregnancy, one in five women experiences spotting.

Painless, small bleeds can be caused by a luteal phase defect. These should have stopped by week 12, 16 at the latest as the placenta fully takes over hormone production at that point.

If the bleeding is due to implantation of the embryo, it should happen a few days before your expected date of the next menstrual period, as the fertilised egg nestles into the uterine lining 4-6 days after fertilisation and the blood from this process takes a few days to make its way to the outside. This bleeding is also light and painless.

Sometimes bleeding can point towards an ectopic pregnancy (between the 6th and 12th week of pregnancy) or a beginning miscarriage. This is mostly accompanied by cramps and/or pain.

A placenta praevia, a placenta that is close to or covers the cervical opening, is also associated with bleeding. Bleeds in later pregnancy are generally caused by placental problems, such as a marginal placental abruption from the wall of the uterus. A placental abruption is a complication sometimes seen after a change in intrauterine pressure or volume. It is usually accompanied with diffuse pain and is a rare complication, often caused by trauma (like a car accident) or intervention (for example an external cephalic version for breech presentation). This can compromise the baby's health acutely.

A definite reason for bleeding can often but not always be found via scan.

In the case of a big fresh bleed up to the 24th week of pregnancy, medicine can generally not do anything to save a potentially compromised baby.

A baby with a compromised blood supply is usually so quiet that the mother either feels reduced movement or none at all, making her concerned about the baby's well being. The justifiably worried mother will go to the doctor or hospital to find out from a scan if her baby is still alive or to birth a baby that has died. If the blood loss is such that the woman is not unduly worried and she does not feel weakened by it, seeking medical attention is not absolutely necessary.

A heavy bleed after 24 weeks is often due to a partial, premature separation of the (sometimes low lying) placenta from the uterine wall. Beyond 24 weeks the chance of a prematurely born baby surviving with the help of modern medicine increases considerably. In that case it is important to attend a hospital that has a neonatal intensive care unit and free space in it.

Before or with onset of contractions for birth, women often have a 'show'. This is usually a light bleed that goes hand in hand with the softening and opening of the cervix and the mucus plug that seals it coming away.

This is usually harmless and heralds the start of labour in the near future.

If you notice a heavy bleed late in pregnancy however (like a continuous trickle) without birth being immediately imminent, you need to seek emergency care straight away as this is a (rare) true emergency.

When pregnancy ends too soon

Miscarriages unfortunately happen and the cause will rarely be found. The woman generally has a bleed, goes to the hospital for a scan to find out if the embryo is still alive or not. If no heartbeat can be found after repeated scans, a dilatation and curettage (D&C) is generally advised.

In my training I have seen the theatre forms for the D&C prepared in the same consultation that confirmed the miscarriage. The woman was not informed of the option to await events and let nature take its course. Hopefully that does not happen in many places anymore.

A D&C is a surgical procedure in which the cervix is opened slowly with dilators that gradually increase in size. Then the contents of the uterus including the uterine lining are scraped out using a sharp spoon like instrument called the curette (hence the procedure being called 'curettage'). The released tissues are then suctioned out of the uterus. The procedure is similar to some abortions up to the 12th week of pregnancy.

Despite it being a routine procedure (that is often done by junior doctors) it is not without dangers. The uterus is much softer due to the hormones of pregnancy and in the worst case scenario, can be perforated or have too much tissue scraped off. In a subsequent pregnancy the placenta may potentially implant into the scar tissue caused by this and have issues with separation after birth. The areas of damage are fortunately not big enough to hinder the birth of the placenta in another pregnancy though.

Studies have not found a connection between placenta accreta (a placenta that is morbidly adhered to the uterine wall and won't separate from the uterine wall after birth) and D&C although it might cause problems in individual cases. (Gielchinsky 2002, Beuker 2005)

It is more likely that a small piece of placenta stays behind in the scarred areas in the uterus, causing increased blood loss after birth (Lohmann-Bigelow 2007). When examining a placenta grown into uterine scar tissue after birth one can often find uterine muscle fibres attached to it. (Jaques 1996)

A D&C should not be performed overly quickly, without careful thought or perhaps with the thought that it is the kindest thing to rid a woman of her dead embryo as quickly as possible. It is important and helpful for a woman's grieving process to take all the time needed to say goodbye to the unborn child.

Normally it is not at all dangerous to await the natural birth of an embryo that has passed away. Even when medical personnel often unlovingly speak of a 'spontaneous abortion' you should be aware of the fact that this is a small birth. Certainly one that has happened far too early, but your body reacts much like it does after a full term birth hormonally. Many women are not prepared for that and often feel very alone when, for example, the milk comes in. A midwife can be very helpful for support and advice. Should there be complications like persistent or heavy bleeding or a temperature you can always seek medical advice.

All this is also relevant when the dead fetus is already bigger. Especially in those fairly rare cases, it seems important for the grieving process to give your body time to let go of the baby naturally.

Women who have already had one or more D&Cs can of course approach pregnancy with confidence despite this. On the whole, apart from a slightly elevated risk of increased blood loss after birth, there are no correlated complications compared to women without a D&C in their history. (Lohmann-Bigelow 2007)

Preparation for birth

What do I need for a self-directed birth?

As already mentioned earlier, you really don't need much for a birth, apart from a pregnant woman and a quiet, warm and dry place – or in case of a waterbirth, a suitable wet place. But there are of course a few helpful **practical things** that most of us already have at home.

Waterproof layers to protect the floor if you are not planning to birth outside or in the pool and a big **towel** to keep the baby dry and warm after birth are amongst them. A **camera** to capture the moment, a **watch** to check time of birth and plenty of food and **drink** are recommended. As food for the post birth period, a good homemade chicken soup is excellent not only for the new mother but also because it can be cooked in a big batch and frozen.

Simple things can make contractions easier, like a warm pool of water (special birthing pools are widely available) in which you can also birth your baby. Alternatively, a normal bathtub will do but is often too small for comfort, a suitable type of water butt is another alternative. Something to lean on or over in hip height (table, washing machine, chest of drawers) or something to hang off (rope, banister or even your partner) can be very soothing for you during contractions. All those little aids can help you explore what makes birth easier for you.

To sever the **cord** (leave about 10 cm of cord attached to the baby) the kitchen scissors will do, to tie it, thread. You can also bite through the cord like other mammals (be patient, it is very tough) and tie off the ends or you simply wait until it falls off by itself, including placenta ('Lotusbirth'), which usually takes between 5 and 10 days. If you have the need to approach this job more professionally, you can order cord clamps on the internet and sterilise some scissors. Studies show that it is beneficial to only sever the cord

once it has ceased pulsing. To avoid issues with the expulsion of the placenta, you should also wait until the placenta has been birthed. Otherwise you can be creative. More about dealing with the cord on page 101.

Most important are a safe, familiar environment and the presence of people you feel comfortable with. This is when the birth hormones flow most easily and most unhindered, particularly oxytocin, and facilitate a straightforward, uncomplicated birth.

If you look at birth in the context of other functions of our pelvic organs, urination, defecation and sex, this is not surprising.

All those processes function similarly. It is not helpful if other people observe your anus closely while you are trying to poop or perhaps even feel how far the faeces have descended in the rectum. Imagine having to do all this while lying on your back. The most likely outcome would be constipation.

It would be equally absurd to try and have sex in a brightly lit room, watched by other people, connected to machines that go beep to measure how close to orgasm you are. As everyone knows, it can be very inhibiting to worry about potential observers during sex. Then imagine someone is constantly checking their watch because they think you should be able to climax in a certain amount of time. Or how about, if you get a couple of minutes in the toilet to finish your business and someone stands in front of the door with a stop watch. You'd probably lose all urge to go.

The only solution to that would probably be to only go to the toilet when it is very nearly too late. This is what some women do when it comes to avoiding a prolonged labour in hospital.

Many birth professionals falsely assume that the cosy atmosphere at home is the irresponsible luxury of an egotistical woman. This is not so. Instead it is of vital importance for a smooth birth.

It is no coincidence that contractions often stop when a woman arrives at the hospital or the midwife arrives (for a homebirth). The hospital is a strange place with strange smells and strange people, and is often connected to unpleasant experiences in the past. All this causes stress. And stress makes the body produce adrenalin, the fight and flight hormone that is in direct opposition to the love and relaxation hormone oxytocin. Who could make love that way? And who feels safe enough to birth the result of love under those circumstances?

Body and soul are closely connected and expecting a woman to birth where she does not feel safe and happy is a direct invitation for complications. Births at home are generally smooth for all the reasons mentioned above. Moreover, things that disturb the finely tuned hormonal interplay of birth don't generally happen at home. Amongst those things are syntocinon drips, induction pessaries and epidurals.

Perineal massage?

Many women fear tears to their perineum, the area between vagina and anus, during birth.

Not long ago it was routine to give all first time mothers a prophylactic episiotomy. These times are not quite over yet as many places still cut episiotomies as soon as a tear seems likely, against all studies and recommendations. (Hartmann & Viswanathan 2005, de Tayrac 2006)

There are many recommendations about the preparation of the perineum for birth: from herbal baths to perineal massage to using a device designed to practice stretching the perineum.

Personally I think this is misguided. The tissues of the perineum don't need preparation to avoid tears. The special cocktail of hormones that is present at the moment of birth is enough to make it appropriately stretchy. Nature did not intend 'pre-stretching' exercises. However, perineal massage may, especially if including your significant other, go some way to alleviate specific fears about perineal tearing.

However, training your pelvic floor (which your perineum is a part of) with frequent squatting and Kegel exercises is certainly recommended. More about that on page 132.

More about tearing and how to avoid it on page 99.

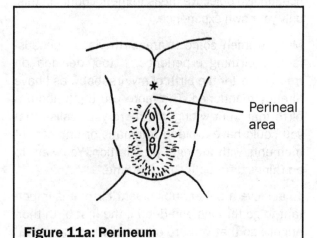

Figure 11a: Perineum
The area between vagina and anus is called the perineum.

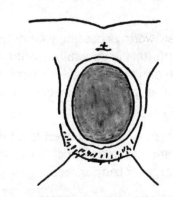

Figure 11b: Perineum during birth
During birth (here on all fours) the perineum gets pushed towards the anus

Traumatic and unpleasant previous birth experiences

A traumatic birth leaves its marks – on the outside as well as on the inside. It often leaves us shocked and hurt. When we get pregnant with the next baby, our big question is usually: Will this happen again?

A birth that was traumatic for the mother did not necessarily look traumatic to bystanders. Finding a birth traumatic or unsatisfactory does not need explanation or justification. No objective measurement counts in this, only your own experience.

Many women come to freebirth via an unsatisfactory birthing experience. I, too, decided on freebirth after the birth of my first baby, as I have already mentioned. The more you think about a birth that went wrong, the more you realise that you could have avoided traumatic or unpleasant moments with the right preparation. You want to do things differently the next time.

To achieve a better subsequent birth, it is important to go through and debrief the first birth thoroughly, so that you are aware of what happened and why. This makes it easier to understand how things went awry and what can go better the next time round. It might also help to get rid of some fears you might be holding on to, justifiably or not.

It is definitely worth accessing your notes from a previous birth (this is generally a written version of your birth and the partogram where dilatation and descent of the baby's head are noted) and copy them or request a copy.

As a patient you are fully entitled to a full copy of your notes and the health trust is legally only allowed to charge for copying fees.

Once you have your notes in your hands, turn to a trusted midwife and go through the birth with her. She will know all the commonly used abbreviations and terminology and can help you understand your records.

You might remember things differently to how they are recorded, or be surprised as to how little or how much time had passed between specific events. The goal is to answer all questions as well as possible and to build up as complete and understandable a picture of the birth as possible. Once you know what went wrong, you can take the next step:

And this is to answer the question as to how you can possibly make your next birth better. This is when you might also start to make peace with what happened.

Practice run in your mind

To prepare for birth, it is useful to play through some scenarios in your mind. You can consider the following:

- What will I do if the birth starts off with my waters breaking but no contractions?
- What will it be like when the contractions start?
- How will I react if things happen very quickly?
- What will I do if I have a long, drawn out birth?
- What if I give birth during the day? Do I want the other children to be present and who will take care of them if I can't?
- What if I can't cope with the contractions?
- When would I potentially call the midwife?
- What will I do if my partner is overwhelmed by something that comes up during birth?

In reality, things might turn out quite differently but practicing different scenarios in your mind can certainly give confidence and can help turn your dream birth into reality.

It is also helpful to think about other coping mechanisms for labour. There is for example Hypnobirthing, a program of meditation and self hypnosis to help with the intensity of contractions ('surges' for the purpose of this program). People who feel Hypnobirthing (there is a book with the same name also) is too time consuming and complicated can still use some of its principles that are also used in other, similar preparation programs.

The most important thing seems to be using your breathing to your advantage. Don't hold your breath but, for example, visualise the opening of your cervix with each breath in and the descent of your baby's head with each breath out. Or breathe the words 'Let (breathe in) go (breathe out)'.

Moreover, singing in low tones can keep you relaxed as a loose lower jaw also leads to a loose pelvic floor. Visualising a blossom opening, the repetition of affirmations, also called birth mantras ('I'm opening wide.') but also distraction and denying labour has actually started can be successful strategies for coping during birth. They can stop you seeing the hard work your body has to do as a threat and help you to surrender to it.

Pain leads to more pain if you try to escape it or even fight it. But if you manage to surrender to it, accept it and bear it with the knowledge that it will bring you closer to your baby, you can make your birth easier and ease the pain with conscious relaxation.

Only one more thing: If you get to the point at which you think you can't do it anymore and none of your strategies seem to bring relief, your baby will likely be born very soon.

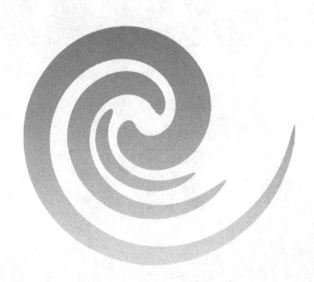

Practical Birth

To start with: good and bad births?

Birth can be a wonderful, life affirming event. For various reasons though, many women nowadays experience their births as humiliating, traumatic and violating. It does not have to be that way and I hope that this book opens doors and enables you to follow your heart and not other people's fears.

It is not my intention to add fire to the flame of envy and competition. Every woman should live her life as she sees fit and birth in the way she feels is right for her. The ability to birth our babies is innate to us, effortlessly. Freebirths are not showing off. Rather they show what is possible when we trust the process of birth and consciously create the optimal environment for our births.

Of course it is possible to make good and bad decisions with regards to birth – it happens all the time, influenced by our experience, fears, circumstances and character. And we should always be careful not to judge others, only because they act, experience and think differently to us.

No mother should ever feel inferior because she didn't manage to have a practically pain free, amazing freebirth. A woman who managed a freebirth with flying colours should never look down on those who didn't manage to or didn't want to. Our backgrounds and lives are just too varied.

Of course there are those – often young and inexperienced in physical things – women who simply go with standard care and have their babies delivered in the hospital and then, when things have not gone to plan, feel grateful they have been 'rescued'.

But honestly, most of us have only become aware of alternatives after negative experiences with mainstream care.

Many women find it difficult facing their fears and happily hand over responsibility for all things to do with pregnancy and birth, and therefore their own bodies, to birth professionals. They push traumatic or abusive experiences during their antenatal care or birth to the back of their mind, and not everyone is strong enough to swim against the tide of societal norms.

Everyone has to live with the consequences of their decisions and we should share our experiences and knowledge to help others make decisions for themselves and their offspring. The more women dare to take the birth of their children into their own hands and talk about it afterwards, the more our voices will be heard.

Every woman who birthed her baby under self direction can help change how society sees pregnant and birthing women. And it is how more and more women realise that there are alternatives to mainstream antenatal and hospital routines.

Apart from medical complications which make a hospital birth necessary, sometimes fear from which a woman cannot free herself makes her choose a hospital birth. We are cultural beings, and doing what is prescribed by our culture and tradition makes us feel safe. We expect certain things to happen because we have always heard and seen it that way. Women who experience a birth (unexpectedly) outside of the hospital, often experience the event as very dramatic and traumatising.

We are culturally conditioned to fear death during birth if we don't birth in the hospital or mimic some of the universally accepted models of care.

How deeply we are conditioned becomes clear by looking at certain YouTube clips: Women who have been moving freely during birth and spent the expulsive phase of labour squatting, suddenly lay down on the floor in the stranded beetle position and let their partners pull out the baby.

However, hospital births that women look back on with joy for the rest of their lives do exist. Sometimes women write to me, tell me about their wonderful, intervention free hospital births and complain that we home and free birthers always connect hospital births with horror and fright.

Of course that isn't the case. Amazing hospital births exist. But looking at the numbers, it becomes clear that birth without interventions are the exception in hospitals and not the norm. In Germany only 8.2% of low risk women have no interventions (Bauer 2010). In contrast, we have a rising caesarean rate of over 30%.

Despite that, many mothers are happy with their hospital births. Even if the birth does not go to plan, expectations (whatever those might be) are fulfilled and that seems enough to satisfy most.

Midwives often report that they encourage women to move around and stay upright during their contractions, but the women prefer to lie on the bed and have an epidural. Those women don't want anything 'newfangled' or natural, but want to birth their babies the way that correlates to their culturally formed view of birth.

Hospital surroundings, with the bed as central point in the room, certainly encourage women to quickly adopt the role of the patient, even if they hadn't planned to. To counteract this, it would be helpful to redesign the layout of hospital rooms and move the immobilising bed into the background.

In terms of physiology, it is without doubt best for mother and baby if a birth happens instinctively without the use of medication and invasive intervention. Some women birth so effortlessly even in the hospital that a birth at home could not possibly have resulted in less intervention.

I'm certainly not in the business to tell happy hospital birthers they should not be happy. If they got what they needed there, who am I to tell them otherwise?

However, women who are unhappy with this standard type of care ought to be aware that there are alternatives. When I released my birth videos on the internet I didn't do so to show women that I could birth better than them. Women have been birthing their babies like that or similarly for millenia.

Every woman is made to birth her babies under her own steam. But society has robbed us of our inner confidence in our bodies and currently we are awfully far from what used to be simply normal for the majority of the history of humankind.

This does not mean that every woman should give birth in a forest or standing up in her living room. The choice of place of birth is a very personal decision, influenced by a variety of different factors. But I would like to show what is possible and widen horizons. We are often so caught up in our cultural humdrum that we are missing out on all the other beautiful paths our lives are offering us.

A completely physiological birth

Textbooks generally distinguish amoung four distinct stages of labour and birth:

- The **first stage of labour** in which the cervix is starting to open.

- Transition.

- The **second stage of labour** during which expulsive contractions help the baby be born.

- During the **third stage of labour** the placenta is expelled.

Being aware of these stages can be helpful, especially if you are aware of what they might feel like. Having said that, eve-

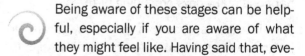

ry birth is different and even after 3 kids, you can still get a surprise during your fourth birth.

By the way, when I talk about contraction, I am not talking about it because it is necessarily connected to pain, but because it is the correct terminology for what is happening, the contraction of the uterine muscle. If you connect contraction with pain, please imagine I am using the word surge.

Here is a short overview over the sensations in each of the phases:

First stage of labour

This often begins several days before the actual birth (prodromal phase) and if a vaginal examination was performed (to be avoided and may cause infection) the cervix would likely be dilated to one or two cm. However, it can still be weeks until proper labour gets going.

In the last few weeks of pregnancy the uterus prepares for birth by contracting now and again. These squeezes (also called Braxton Hicks contractions) make the uterus go noticeably hard and can sometimes even be painful.

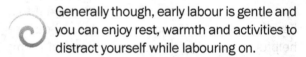 It is sometimes hard to know what are practice contractions and what is the real thing. Even regular contractions can disappear again completely and start up again a few days later.

A sign of labour likely to start soon is the loss of the mucus plug, or **show**, which appears when the neck of the womb shortens and begins to open. It is a slimy, often bloody glob of mucus which closes off the cervix throughout the whole pregnancy (protecting the fetus from ascending bacteria from the vagina), and it often comes away shortly before birth – though sometimes it happens many days preceding birth.

For all these reasons it is quite easy to wrongly judge the start of labour. A very definitive sign for

an imminent labour is your **waters breaking**. Although only a small proportion of births starts off with a 'proper rupture of membranes'.

There is also something called a '**hind water leak**' which means the amniotic sac has a small hole higher up in the uterus or a 'false' rupture of membranes where one of the two layers of amniotic sac break. Both of these events generally only release a small amount of amniotic fluid and birth can still be a long way off.

In the days before birth, you often experience a bit of **diarrhea**. It seems like your body wants to get rid of any sort of ballast and clear the way for the baby. But this can also happen without labour being imminent.

The start of labour can be very intense, making you wake up suddenly in the middle of the night, jumping out of bed and wondering how you can cope with a labour this intense if this is only the beginning. If the birth is not extremely fast and the baby is not born shortly after a sudden start like this, labour may mellow out again and lessen in pain levels and intensity.

Generally though, early labour is gentle and you can enjoy rest, warmth and activities to distract yourself while labouring on.

Because you never know how long labour is going to last, it is a good idea to continue doing what you were planning on doing anyway.

During the night, that means sleeping, even if that means in 15 or 20 minute increments between contractions.

During the day or when lying down in bed is not possible anymore, getting on with some everyday activities is a great way to get you through early labour.

Frequent visits to the toilet can be very helpful as your bowels and bladder can freely clear themselves out. If your waters have gone, it can make sense to actively get rid of amniotic fluid (perhaps by circling your pelvis over the toilet) so that the uterus can recognise the change in volume and contract efficiently.

Many women tidy up in the first stage of labour, clean, prepare their place of birth and get their partner to fill the pool. They might also get really hungry or organise care for older children if present. With time, contractions become more intense and require lots of attention and possibly leaning over the washing machine, chest of drawers or kitchen table.

Towards the end of the first stage of labour, many women pace the floor, completely within themselves, ready for the next contraction, that likely will require breathing through or vocalising. The contractions get closer and closer, become more intense and then birth merges seamlessly into ...

Transition

Now contractions seem on top of each other. Powerful, and possibly relentless. Mentally, if the birth has been undisturbed, women tend to be very much in their own world at this point, but at the same time very present with what is happening. Every contraction requires huge concentration but still they become more frequent and don't give many breaks.

Breathing, singing, vocalising, holding on ... everything that helped up to now doesn't particularly help anymore. Women are often restless between contractions and mobilise a lot.

This is the classic point at which women often say or think things like: 'I don't want to do this anymore, I can't.' 'Make it stop.' 'Take me to the hospital, I want a caesarean!' or 'I'm going to die if this doesn't stop soon.'

These feelings are quite existentialist and you often really do feel for a moment that you might die. This phase of birth is the most difficult, mentally and physically. You reach the end of your strength, but at the same time you go beyond the strength you thought you had. Your legs shake, you are cold and hot at the same time and some women vomit. It is easy to tense up and pull up your shoulders at this time, but it is important to remind yourself to relax.

This is also the point during which well placed humour can come to the rescue. When I got to this phase during my first freebirth, truly alone and in the forest, in the midst of my 'misery', the song 'Silent Night' suddenly popped into my head. I began to sing and the lyrics were on the one hand so fitting for my situation but on the other hand so absurd that I began to laugh and relaxed at the same time.

The good thing about this difficult transition phase is the fact that you have come so far that it is nearly over. Because right after it, the irresistible urge to push out the baby sets in.

Second stage of labour

The urge to push only sets in when the baby's head is nicely tucked into the pelvis and touches a certain spot. So you don't particularly have to think about how dilated your cervix is.

Some women do feel their cervix in labour to reassure themselves of progress, but others don't feel the need or can't actually reach their cervix.

Cervical dilatation is a misleading diagnostic parameter, clinically. Some women are fully dilated in the hospital but have no urges to push, yet are urged to do so. In this situation it is likely that the baby's head is in a suboptimal position – and therefore does not cause the urge to push yet. Premature pushing can result in problems that are often solved with various interventions.

If the urges to push just don't seem to start though, you could try a little push to see what happens. During my first birth the midwife suggested this and it made the urge appear promptly. As soon as pushing is inevitable, the challenges of transition are overcome. The woman knows that she has nearly done it. Soon the little head can be felt and you just want to get it over with. However, out of politeness towards your perineum, taking it slowly might be a better idea.

Crowning of the baby's head and also the birth of the shoulders, can be unpleasant – or even pleasant and orgasmic, as the baby's body sliding and turning through the cervix is a sensation without comparison – but then the baby's body is already born and the rush of happy hormones makes us forget our efforts.

Don't be surprised though if there is a little break between the birth of the baby's head and the rest of the body. This is quite normal as the body waits for the rotation of the shoulders to occur.

Please don't tug at the head in this situation (as it is often done during 'managed' births) or push excessively. Give your body – and the baby's body – the time it needs. (More on page 90, 'What if ... there is a shoulder dystocia?'

Third stage of labour

While the mother greets her baby, the baby latches and they both take a breather from the efforts of birth, the placenta detaches from the wall of the uterus, is born gently and without pain. Normally this happens at some point during the hour after birth.

If you want, after an instinctive period of waiting, you can try to pull on the cord and gently push out the placenta. If the **placenta** has already detached, this is easy and painfree. If not, wait some more.

Once the placenta is expelled, it's a good time to cut the cord.

'Rest and be thankful' phase

The 'rest and be thankful' phase is very important for experienced midwives. This is a phase that happens in the first stage of labour or shortly before the second stage and is marked by – as appears on the outside – nothing much happening at all.

Contractions become weaker, the breaks become longer and sometimes it seems like the mother's body is contemplating if it wants to carry on with labour or not. Before the second stage of labour this is usually called 'the calm before the storm'. It is like the subconscious has to catch up with the physical body and give its consent to end the pregnancy and start a new life with a newborn.

This phase requires patience and time and should not be rushed by medical intervention. Birth is not always a linear, predictable event, and a 'rest and be thankful' phase is no indication for intervention.

Birth on land

As already mentioned, staying upright and mobile are incredibly beneficial to encourage a straightforward birth.

Not only because gravity and mobility enable the mother to help the baby find its way – which includes rotation – but also because at the time the baby passes through the pelvis, the mother's **sacrum** and **coccyx** move out of the baby's way.

This movement makes more room for the baby but also makes the maternal pelvis somewhat unstable so that the mother often feels like holding on to something.

Being on her back or sitting hinders the pelvis in expanding as wide as possible. It also prohibits circling pelvic movement or similar to help the baby rotate through the pelvis. These positions are the most frequent reasons for non progressing labour and difficult birth that prompt epidurals and instrumental births.

Standing, **squatting** or **kneeling** are ideal in this regard as they provide the baby with all the available room in the pelvis.

I'm often asked if I wasn't afraid to drop the baby when birthing standing up all by myself. Funnily enough I never thought about that during the birth. I just did what I had to do. I do know of some women who didn't feel able to catch their own babies. The partner can always do it or you can always bolster the floor with an air mattress or soft cushions.

We shouldn't be too afraid of the possibility of the baby dropping to the ground though. Babies are quite robust and likely don't come to harm, should it happen. Animal mothers don't catch their young and some, for example giraffes, tend to fall quite a distance.

I do in fact know of a mother who dropped her baby in the shower. The cord snapped, there was blood everywhere but the baby was just fine. Of course I am not saying you should drop your baby on purpose, but you shouldn't avoid birthing standing up if it feels right because of those fears.

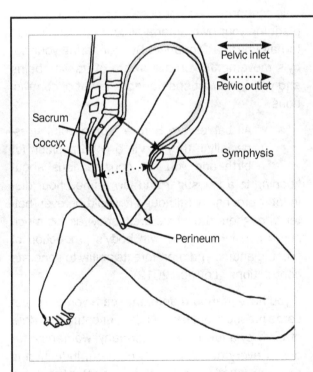

Figure 12a: Upright birthing position
In an upright position both sacrum and coccyx have room to move. The baby has all the room it needs to pass through the pelvis. In addition, gravity helps.

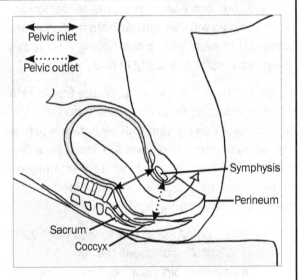

Figure 12b: Semi recumbent (half sitting) birthing position
The semirecumbent woman sits/lies on her sacrum and coccyx. There is only limited movement, the baby may have difficulty moving through the pelvis. The baby is pushed in an upward curve to be born.

Notice the increased strain on the perineum.

Birth in water

Many women love birthing in water. The warm water relieves the powerful sensations of labour and, of course, the baby can be born in the water too. The water temperature should be comfortable to you. To get the best relaxation benefits from being in the water, the water level should at least reach to just above your bump when sitting, ideally even higher.

If you get into the pool in early labour it is possible that your contractions will lessen and labour slows down. This can also be a sign that labour had not started properly yet and many midwives use it as a test to see if labour is established or not.

As a rule, you should get in the pool as late as possible, but every woman needs to decide for herself and go with her gut. Warmth and calm are beneficial in early labour and having a bath can be just as helpful as staying in bed.

If a baby is born into a warm pool, the first breath is only stimulated when it reaches (cool) air. Getting the baby into contact with air before it is fully born should therefore be avoided. Due to the fact that there is less or rather different stimulation for the baby, breathing is often initiated a little more slowly than during land births.

When giving Apgar scores (see page 124) one should not count the time from the moment of birth but from the moment of leaving the water. But officially, the time of birth remains as the moment when that last part of the baby emerges from the mother's body (excluding placenta and umbilical cord).

It is possible to rent birthing pools for waterbirths at home, and some women also use a normal paddling pool as well as their bath, if big enough. As a space saving alternative, a big rain water butt can also be used, with a stool on the inside and outside to make getting in and out easier.

What if ...

On the following pages I want to answer a few questions that tend to come up automatically when thinking about freebirth.

Please keep in mind that I am approaching these answers from a homebirth and self direction point of view. In hospitals, deviations from the norm can have other reasons, often caused by intervention or environment. Procedures to deal with certain scenarios may also be different, due to strict protocols in hospital.

But what happens if I am birthing my baby by myself and ...

... I am overdue?

This scenario does not pose a problem if you are planning your own antenatal care and don't wish to have birth attendance. By monitoring your baby's movements you are aware of its well being and you can await spontaneous onset of contractions.

All babies are born at some point – especially if they are in a good position for birth and you are conscientious about keeping to a low sugar and low refined flour diet in later pregnancy (although it would be even better throughout the whole pregnancy) as too much sugar can inhibit your own body's production of prostaglandins and therefore its ability to generate contractions. (Louwen 2012)

If you have standard antenatal care you often get some pressure once you pass your estimated date of birth by a few days. In Germany, women go for a CTG every two days from then on, induction is recommended from about 7 days after the dates and strongly recommended at 14 days late.

It is common practice to do ultrasound scans to check on the baby's well being. Often a 'calcified' placenta and 'low levels of amniotic fluid' are identified and the pregnant woman is told that her baby really needs to be born.

What they don't tend to tell you is that some calcification in the placenta and a lowering of amniotic fluid levels are rather normal towards the end of pregnancy. Many midwives supporting homebirths are only happy to do so until 12 to 14 days past the EDB. Women who have not birthed their babies by then and are left by their midwife need to go to the hospital or have a freebirth. In the UK however, women have a right to a midwife attending their homebirth, no matter how far past their due date they are.

If you have ruled out a possible mistake calculating the due date (maybe due to delayed ovulation) you have every reason to stay relaxed and not let the birth professionals worry you. A normal pregnancy lasts 40 weeks +/- 2 weeks. This means that a baby going past its due date by 14 days is still within normal parameters.

And of course there are women who just have longer pregnancies and always go far over their dates. A big study has concluded that the vast majority of births happen within 3 weeks before EDB and 3 weeks after. (Jukic 2013)

Women who accept induction sometimes believe that their body cannot produce contractions by itself. But the ones who have the courage to await events, simply birth after a longer pregnancy. To counteract this stress, lots of women, particularly the ones who have already experienced a longer pregnancy and the stresses associated with that, simply state the date of their last menstrual period as 1 to 2 weeks later than it actually was.

Maybe I should also mention that many investigations suggest a normal pregnancy lasts closer to 283 days rather than 280 days as previously assumed (Bergsjö et al 1990, Smith 2001) and that the calculations of Boerhave from 1744 may have been interpreted wrongly. He talks about 'nine month after the last menstrual period' but does not mention if he means the beginning or the end of the period. Potentially he was talking about the end and not the beginning which would account for the extra 3 days more recent studies have found.

As long as your gut tells you it is ok and your baby is moving well, don't let them worry you. Don't go where people put pressure on you and disappear into your little pregnancy bubble. Your patience may be put to the test but on the scale of things, what difference will a few days make after the many months of pregnancy? Your baby will start labour in collaboration with your body, once you are both ready for it.

Sometimes the baby's awkward positioning can prevent engagement into the pelvis. And as' long as the baby is not in an optimal position for birth, labour can be delayed. This delay is sometimes accompanied by runs of painful contractions as your body's attempts to coax the baby into a better position. These bouts of discomfort often rob the mother of strength and sleep. This tends to go on as long as it takes to get the baby into a good position or until the birth professional's patience, or often the mother's patience, runs out and birth is induced pharmaceutically.

In cases of suboptimal fetal positioning (or fetal malpositioning) birth can truly be overdue. If you suspect that your baby is in a less than optimal position, there are certain exercises you can do to move the baby into a better position, as described on page 60. There is also the possibility that certain areas in the baby's brain or lungs are still not developed enough to signal the start of labour.

Attempting to artificially start labour with castor oil (also called castor oil cocktail or midwife's cocktail) is absolutely not recommended in this context.

It might seem tempting, because it sounds like a completely natural way to induce. However, keep your hands off as you never know how your immune system may react. In the best case scenario, nothing happens or labour starts and goes ahead without problems. Worst case scenario, castor oil can stimulate a massive histamine response from your immune system, leading to maternal collapse or placental abruption – which puts your baby in mortal danger.

... the baby is big?

This fear is a very modern problem and often due to obese and malnourished mothers but mostly a problem created by overzealous ultrasound use. Of course big babies that are more difficult to birth than normal sized babies (around 3.000g, 50cm long) do exist too.

However, you can avoid an abnormally large baby by keeping your blood sugars levels even, either by diet or, in the case of serious pregnancy diabetes, with medication such as insulin.

Back to the ultrasound oracle: By measuring the length of bones and physical circumferences, a computer calculates estimated body weight – and is often hopelessly wrong. Discrepancies of up to a kilo are not rare. And still, decisions to induce and perform caesarean sections are made on the basis of these measurements.

If you want a better estimation of weight, let an experienced midwife feel your belly. Midwives are often very good at precise estimations of birth weight, due to their experience. Precise in this context means: Small/medium/large in relation to the mother. The exact number of grams is not really important.

And what if the baby really is too big? Well, it might make the birth more difficult and exhausting but ultimately, with an upright posture and plenty of time, definitely doable. The baby's head remains the largest diameter to pass through the pelvis and it simply does not grow much in the last few days before birth so that 'moving the birth forward' by induction (if indeed it works) is not a good alternative. If the head can pass through the pelvis, the rest of the body follows.

There is not much difference between a small and a big baby's head because the fat is generally spread over the rest of the body. And even if the baby's tummy is particularly podgy: fat squishes and will fit through somehow. It is not as hard as a boney head.

Mind you, the baby's head is not all that hard either, but actually very flexible and resembles a patchwork blanket due to the fontanels. This is how the parts of the baby's skull can slide over each other and mould through tight spaces.

A cone headed baby is the result of our body's brilliant ability to adapt, and of course the odd shape will be gone before the first hat needs to be tried for size.

... my waters break but contractions don't start immediately?

A true rupture of membranes generally heralds the start of labour, and usually contractions start shortly after. Especially if the mother – as described above – empties as much amniotic fluid into the toilet as possible, to stimulate the uterus into contracting. But it is certainly possible for nothing to happen initially. Then you can wait.

In most cases, labour will start within 24 hours and the baby will be born within 48 hours. As long as you are well, don't have a temperature or other signs of an ascending infection, you don't have to worry about labour not starting immediately.

Vaginal examinations should be avoided in the waiting period to stop the introduction of bacteria. Even if you lost a lot of amniotic fluid, your baby is not in 'on dry land' now. Amniotic fluid is regenerated all the time and probably washes out potential germ, away from the uterus and baby. If you still don't feel any contractions after 24 hours, putting in a probiotic vaginal supplement (as mentioned previously) to guard against infection, may be sensible. Sometimes the amniotic fluid comes from a small tear in the amniotic sac and can reseal itself, in which case the leak was probably small rather than torrential.

Of course it is also possible to confuse a leak of urine from the bladder with a rupture of membranes. A test strip to determine pH-value, such as litmus paper can show up liquor, which is alkaline. The vagina is usually acidic. However, urine can also be alkaline, depending on what you have been eating.

So litmus paper is not reliable to distinguish between urine and amniotic fluid. You can however use your nose and touch to distinguish between the two: Amniotic fluid smells quite different to urine, more fruity-aromatic and feels rather silky and slippery.

... I go into labour too soon?

Sometimes the question of when it might be safe to stay at home with regards to gestation, and when the baby may need medical support after a premature birth, comes up.

By definition, babies born before the completed 37th week of pregnancy are classed as premature. Generally, midwives are unwilling to support such a birth. The earlier the birth, the more support the newborn usually requires.

A premature baby (I am not referring to very premature babies, but to the ones born after 3o weeks of pregnancy) has an underdeveloped respiratory system and often has trouble regulating its temperature, especially if the birth was sudden and without many practice contractions which stimulate lung maturation. Another issue can be increased jaundice levels and difficulties suckling, but those are not necessarily problematic immediately after birth, but rather after a few days.

It is important to stop a premature baby from overheating or cooling, and keeping it skin to skin with the mother. The mother wearing seasonally appropriate clothes or blankets (if she is in her bed) over her and the baby is the best way to achieve this. Another thing to keep an eye on is humidity. Dry air can make it more difficult for the immature lungs to absorb oxygen. If the air seems too dry, getting into a warm bathroom with a hot shower running so that the air is nice and humid (achieved when the mirror is all steamed up) can be helpful.

However, there are big differences in maturity from baby to baby. Some are absolutely fine to breathe normal air without help from 34 weeks while others still struggle to breathe unaided after two more weeks of gestation.

If birth happens at borderline gestation, I feel it is justifiable to still birth at home and await how the baby adapts. If in any doubt, call a doctor or midwife to ask for advice and use the tricks above to help.

Should the baby show any issues with adaptation to extrauterine life that need treatment, there should be enough time to go to hospital.

Babies with an immature respiratory system don't tend to struggle straight away, but tire easily and find breathing more and more difficult. One sign to look out for is the use of auxiliary respiratory muscles by the newborn. Its small body utilises all its strength to get enough oxygen. You can observe sucking in of the muscles between the ribs (intercostals) and the flaring of the nostrils, all in the rhythm of respiration.

Even when the baby is born at term it can show the same signs of an immature respiratory system in the context of delayed adaptation to extrauterine life, and may be so busy breathing that it is unable to suckle. These difficulties generally ease quickly, as soon as the baby breathes humidified air. If there is no relief, it is sensible to seek medical attention.

... contractions are painful but labour does not progress?

The reason for this is usually a malpositioned fetal head, that is not optimally engaged into the pelvis. To be able to engage, the baby needs to turn its head to look towards one side of the mother's pelvis.

Normally, the baby puts its chin on its chest while engaging. If it doesn't, this move becomes more difficult or, in some situations, impossible.

While malpositioned, the baby's head pushes against the mother's sacrum, causing strong back pain during or even between contractions.

The birthing mother often finds counterpressure very helpful but counterpressure alone can be counterproductive unless she changes her own position as well. This is because the back pain is signaling a malposition and shows that the baby requires more room in the pelvis to turn, yet the counterpressure makes less room.

If the head is not turned to the side to engage into the pelvis, swinging and circling the hips and gently shaking your bottom can encourage a better position. If the head has already entered the pelvis (perhaps with its head in a neutral position and not with the chin on the chest), you can provide an opportunity to disengage and then engage again in a better position by resting your hips higher than your upper body (see knee chest position, page 62) for about 3 contractions while circling your hips and shaking your bottom.

The high hips enable the baby to move out of the pelvis again by utilising gravity. This stretches the uterine ligaments, there is more room in the pelvis and the baby can re-engage in a more fitting way (Tully 2012).

Walking up and down the stairs sideways is another way to help the fetal head into a more optimal position.

Should you also have a 'stargazer' on board, it is still possible for it to turn during these maneuvers. See more about turning such a baby on page 59.

Everything that potentially reduces room in the pelvis for the baby to turn is counterproductive at this point. The woman often has the instinctive urge to make her back hollow. This can also widen the pelvic inlet. In the hospital, women often sit in a hospital bed at this time in their labour, making it impossible for the sacrum to move back and provide room. Perhaps this is one of the reasons for the increase in posterior, stargazing babies.

As a freebirther you may not necessarily know exactly how your baby is positioned, so I would recommend first elevating and circling your hips and then doing the same in an upright position.

In practice, always be led by your body. Although I didn't know anything about exercises helping with positioning, instinctively I was doing the right movements for me anyway and circled my hips which eventually helped my baby's head to get into a good position.

How long you carry on without success is up to you. At the latest, the point at which the mother's strength is fading is a good time to seek professional advice.

Another specific problem can be **deep one sided pain in your pelvis**. This is often due to the baby's head being in an **asynclitic position**, which means it is tilted towards one of its shoulders.

To solve this problem and to get the baby into the pelvis, the following exercises in addition to the ones above can be helpful:

- Climbing stairs

- Swinging your hips sideways and elevating them on one side

- Resting with one foot higher than the other (perhaps on a stool or stack of books) – you will likely know which foot to elevate instinctively

- tilting your pelvis during contractions

Another reason for one sided pelvic pain can be a compound presentation, which is usually a **hand in front or by the side** of the baby's head.

Following measures can coax the hand away from the head:

- kneel on one knee

- swinging the hips forward, first on one side, then the other, while bending the knees and standing on tiptoes.

- a vaginal examination (you can of course do that yourself if you wish) and touching or pressing on the baby's fingertips can make it retract the hand (Sutton 2010)

... there is a cord prolapse?

A cord prolapse is a very rare, but potentially life threatening situation for the baby. It occurs when the cord gets trapped between the baby's head, bottom (breech presentation) or body (transverse lie) and the cervix.

The danger here is that the pressure to the cord cuts off the baby's blood supply and starves it of oxygen if it can't counteract this pressure by upping blood pressure sufficiently.

If there is a cord prolapse you can generally feel a soft pulsating mass next to the baby's hard head or relatively firm bottom while doing a vaginal examination. A loop of cord might extend into the vagina or even protrude from it.

An effective emergency measure is elevating the hips higher than the upper body (knee chest position, page 62). This takes unnecessary pressure off the cord as the baby's head moved off the cervix, which makes it potentially possible to free the cord and push it back up into the uterus and process with a normal birth. This should however not be done alone but with an experienced midwife in attendance.

If this fails, and the baby can not be born quickly, you should go to hospital immediately, either with elevated hips or lying on your side.

You don't have to worry about cord prolapse if your baby is normally positioned and has already engaged into the pelvis in preparation for birth. Cord prolapse is more common in premature births, multiple births and breech birth, particularly if a loop of cord is already positioned near the cervix.

With the latter, the cord does not generally get squeezed shut completely as the soft presenting parts, like bottom and legs enable the blood to keep flowing.

Another scenario that raises the risk for cord prolapse is the presence of abnormally large amounts of amniotic fluid, the cord is particularly long or your membranes are ruptured artificially without the baby descending into the pelvis.

We don't know if the risk is also elevated if the baby's head has not engaged in the pelvis at the start of labour. (Murphy 1998, Debby 2003)

In German speaking countries, women are often advised to lay down immediately when their waters break and call an ambulance. There is no evidence for the benefit of this and is unheard of in other countries.

Some speculate that this protocol may even increase the risk for cord prolapse. When the cord is washed down as the water breaks, it happens slowly because it is not very dense and fairly light. The baby's head is much heavier and more dense and moves much faster, not giving the cord a chance to reach the cervix first.

Generally, the baby's head will drop onto the cervix immediately after the waters break to plug the leak, so to say. If you still have concerns, you can feel your belly carefully for the head and see if it seems firmly plugged in the pelvis, hugged tightly by the lower segment of the uterus or is still movable over the symphysis pubis.

You can also feel via the vagina if the head is tightly engaged or is still easily pushed out of the pelvis with your fingers.

The risk for cord prolapse is only around 0.3%, even including premature births, artificial rupture of membranes etc and is therefore very low (Koonings 1990, Kahana 2004, Boyle 2005). This is quite disproportionate to the fear many women hold of this emergency.

... I have an anterior lip of cervix, like I did during a previous birth?

Sometimes the midwife can feel a lip of cervix once the cervix is nearly all the way open. Often women are told not to push until the lip is gone. A midwife can massage or push such a lip of cervix

away if it is causing pain or becomes swollen. This is generally very painful for women.

So, what about this ominous lip of cervix? The cervix does not open as an even circle as it is generally illustrated in textbooks, rather more like an oval depending on the shape of the baby's head and from the back to the front, yielding to the pressure of the head (see illustr 13).

So the last bit of opening happens at the front, particularly if a previous caesarean scar is present.

On the whole, the presence of an anterior cervical lip is quite normal for a certain amount of time. But this last bit of cervix left to open can cause pain and discomfort, especially if the baby's head, which plays a huge role for the opening of the cervix, is not optimally positioned. A woman can even push this lip of cervix away herself, easiest on all fours. It is located at the front of the vagina, right behind the symphysis pubis.

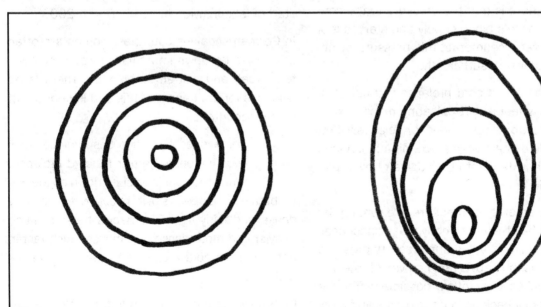

Figure 13: Opening of the cervix during birth from 0 to 10 cm
On the left, theoretical progress, on the right, actual progress.

... there is fetal distress and I don't notice?

There are various reasons why a baby might be compromised in utero during or even before birth, resulting in abnormal heart rate.

Unfortunately the monitoring of the baby's heartbeat via a CTG (cardiotocograph) machine often leads even experienced birth professionals on the wrong path and has unfortunately not improved safety during birth. Quite the opposite: a CTG monitoring is far too inaccurate to evaluate fetal well being. The only thing it has value for is checking the presence and absence of a fetal heart beat, everything in between is like an oracle.

No cardiologist would feel confident evaluating the condition of a heart patient, just by looking at a tracing of the heart beat. The current reliance on the heart rate tracing from the CTG machine is likely one of the main reasons for the increasing caesarean rate.

The most important and reliable measure of the baby's well being is the woman's perception of her baby's spontaneous and reactive movements. Women can feel those without technology and they are more reliable than CTGs.

But you should know that the baby's heart rate does not simply deteriorate suddenly. Generally this requires an induced labour or an abnormally long and arduous one (perhaps due to the position the mother is in) that leads the baby to inadequate use of glucose or an electrolyte imbalance.

Other reasons for abnormal heart tracings and distress in the baby can be other interventions, or perhaps a pathology in the baby, such as a malformation of the cord and/or placenta.

Often the baby's heart rate slows in a compensatory manner for a few moments towards the end of labour or becomes difficult to listen to, which often leads to rush and panic in a hospital environment.

However it is within normal parameters for the baby to show a slowing of its heart rate for a short time due to the strain of the expulsive contractions in the second stage of labour. The stress that often goes hand in hand with this in the hospital is generally of no benefit to anyone and the mother often ends up with a syntocinon drip or other intervention which does nothing to alleviate the baby's potential distress.

... there is meconium?

Meconium stained amniotic fluid is not a sign of distress in the baby by itself (Unsworth & Vause 2010) but can be an indicator for distress in combination with other signs. Thick meconium in liquor is more likely to be a problem than light meconium staining.

As everyone knows, babies pass urine in utero but the mother's body is very good at fluid exchange and soon the amniotic fluid is clean again. Babies only tend to poo once they are born, but not always. Especially babies that are past their EDB sometimes do their first poo in utero.

When your **amniotic fluid is stained green**, there are three possibilities:

1.) perhaps the baby pooped because it is stressed or afraid

2.) it needed a poo

3.) the normal stress of labour prompted the baby to poop

Only a small percentage of babies remains distressed after pooing in utero.

Further action would depend on how labour has proceeded so far and I would ask myself the following questions:

- Is this birth going well or are there any abnormalities?
- Is the baby moving adequately and does it seem well?
- What is the mother's gut feeling?

When meconium is present in the amniotic fluid, birth professionals are also worried about another rare complication. Occasionally a distressed baby inhales meconium in the liquor and an infection can result (meconium aspiration syndrome). This is potentially life threatening for the baby but very rare. Only a very distressed baby inhales meconium.

Meconium in the fluid around the baby therefore does not present danger by itself, but becomes an issue when the baby is so distressed that it attempts to gasp for air in utero. So you should avoid everything that is likely to stress the baby, such as: induction or artificial augmentation of labour, artificial rupture of membranes, stress for the mother (which can decrease blood flow through the placenta), coached 'purple pushing' etc etc.

... the shoulders get stuck?

This happens in approximately 1% of births. The head is born, but the shoulders don't rotate to be born but get stuck behind the mother's pubic bone. Birth professionals sometimes also call this 'sticky shoulders' or shoulder dystocia. You can pretty much rule this out if you don't have diabetes, are not significantly obese, don't have a larger than average baby on board (often connected with maternal diabetes), have not been induced with syntocinon, don't have a vacuum extraction, don't birth lying on your back or sitting on your bottom and don't get coached to push.

The best prophylaxis is good nutrition and the avoidance of intervention common in hospital as well as good birthing positions. Should the shoulders get stuck despite all this, getting into all fours is often enough to dislodge them. (Gaskin 1998)

Another possibility is to push the stuck shoulder to one side so that the shoulders can be born, one after the other. (Rockel-Loenhoff 2010)

... the cord is around baby's neck?

The fear of the umbilical cord is strong in modern obstetrics. It is seriously believed that babies, perhaps from boredom or by coincidence, might strangle themselves with it.

If a cause for a non progressing labour or the sudden death of a baby in utero cannot be found, the cord is generally the scapegoat. And because the cord is wrapped around the baby's neck at least once in about a third of all births, this seems a reasonable assumption.

However, a cord wrapped around the baby's neck, however many times, is not an emergency in reality. The baby does not need to breathe yet and is supplied with oxygen from maternal blood from the wrapped (but not occluded) cord and therefore can't suffocate.

How is it possible that the cord still works, even if it is wrapped tightly? It is designed from such a material and in such a way that it can be pulled hard and wrapped tight without losing much of its function. Blood flow might reduce momentarily, but a baby will still receive some and recover quickly from a short lack of oxygen supply during birth.

A short or wrapped cord doesn't stop the baby from being born either as the uterus, including placenta and cord follow the baby during its descent into the pelvis.

The baby is not like a lamp hanging from the ceiling and requires a certain length of cord to be able to exit the uterus. Due to the uterus directly following the baby's bottom as it is pushed into and through the pelvis, there is always enough slack for the baby to come out. As soon as the head is born, the baby can take a breath if need be.

So what should you do if you can see that the cord is wrapped round the baby's neck?

In the hospital, cords often get unraveled even before the baby's body is born. Even though this only takes seconds it can lead to a 'strangling re-flex' (a carotid sinus syncope is triggered with the associated drop in heart rate and blood pressure) and should therefore be avoided.

Rough handling of the cord can furthermore lead to a reflexive constriction of the vessels within it.

It is better to just leave the cord in peace. Babies tend to be born perfectly fine with the cord round their necks. Once they are born, you can unravel the cord.

... the baby doesn't breathe?

It is quite normal for the baby to take some time to transition from not breathing in the womb to active breathing in the outside world. This is be-cause the lungs, which have never actively worked before, have to switch to a new type of circulation to activate. This happens immediately or a short time after birth.

For this reason the apgar score is not evaluated until one minute after birth, 5 minutes after birth and sometimes again after 10 and 60 minutes. This concludes that newborns take a few minutes to 'arrive' properly, with some being present and breathing immediately and some needing a little longer to come round.

During birth, the baby's body goes through a series of complex processes of which we only really see the onset of breathing from the outside. A baby who is not breathing yet is still supplied with oxygen, as long as the cord is pulsing and blood is pumped from placenta to baby.

Certain biochemical processes help stop this blood flow and the baby initiates breathing to ac-tively supply himself with oxygen. In some free-birth videos you can see the tension and fear that arises if a baby is not breathing immediately and even appears to be floppy in its mother's arms.

Generally, it does not take longer than a minute until the baby reacts to outside stimulus. But even if the cord is still puls-ing, waiting for that very first breath can make sec-onds feel like a very long time. Gentle stimulation like stroking, soft rubbing or blowing into the ba-by's face are often enough to encourage the baby to breathe.

Most babies are slightly purple or blue at birth but become pink in the first few minutes. They have good muscle tone and soon start respirations.

Some babies keep the purple-bluey colour in their face while the rest of the body is nice and pink. This is generally harmless and due to venous congestion from birth. Hands and feet can also remain somewhat blue for a few hours after birth. This is also harmless and occurs frequently.

Then there are babies who need more time. Perhaps they take a few breaths and have good muscle tone but then stop breathing and become floppy. You should keep stimulating such a baby and check the cord is pulsing. Usually it is.

If mucus or amniotic fluid is present in the nose or mouth, you can suck it out with your mouth or a nose aspirator for newborns. If the baby does not respond to suctioning, you can start mouth to nose resuscitation.

In the book 'Emergency Childbirth' anoth-er method for resuscitation is described: One hand holds the baby's hips, the other the upper body and head. Then you move your hands in such a way that knees and upper body come together, about 12 times per minute. (White 1998)

The folding movement compresses the baby's lungs and air escapes, while the stretching out lets them expand and the negative pressure en-courages a repeated filling of the lungs.

What makes it more likely for a baby to take its time with breathing? Premature babies, babies who have trouble with blood sugar regulation and babies with an infection are more likely to have issues with the transition to breathing independently.

In the hospital, certain drugs make this transition more difficult, for example pethidine (analgesia) or benzodiazepines (tranquilisers). Caesarean babies may also struggle with this issue as well as babies who have certain severe abnormalities incompatible with breathing and in some cases life.

From the many birth stories I have read, it becomes clear that most mothers instinctively know how to support their babies at birth. And they are also the ones who know when everything is ok, even when there is no one else around.

I do know a few birth stories in which a baby was born floppy and slow to breathe. All of those eventually recovered well and had a good start in life, either with resuscitation by their mother or a midwife and without a doctor's attention.

In some cases, panicked fathers called an ambulance and traumatic days followed for mother and baby in the hospital or neonatal intensive care unit, not because there was something seriously wrong, but because the babies were born at home which was considered a danger in itself.

In other cases a midwife was called and the problem was solved in a calm manner.

Even if such a start seems like quite the shock: you shouldn't expect a full term, healthy baby to have lasting difficulties with breathing at birth. A healthy baby can generally withstand even a stressful birth.

... the baby inhales some of the amniotic fluid?

During its time in utero the baby has practiced breathing. But what did it breathe in? Nothing. It only exercised its diaphragm to be able to manage its first breath when born. For this, the baby doesn't need the fluid produced in the lungs anymore.

Helpfully the baby's chest will be compressed while passing through the maternal pelvis and pelvic floor and has most of the fluid squeezed out of it in the process.

Babies born by caesarean section miss out on this squeeze and sometimes encounter problems with their breathing.

A natural birth eliminates most of this lung fluid but some generally remains. This is why newborns often breathe quite noisily, which is quite normal.

The remaining liquid is absorbed by the lungs, after which breathing noise usually fades (after about 20 minutes) and then disappears.

In hospitals, the newborn's stomach is sometimes suctioned, due to the misguided belief that firstly, it will eliminate the fluid that causes the noise and secondly to rule out an esophageal atresia. Because unless you actively try to put the suction tube into the trachea for intubation with the help of a laryngoscope, you generally end up in the esophagus.

Esophageal atresia is a rare malformation in which the esophagus either has a very narrow passage or a dead end.

An examination to rule this out can however still be performed if there is a suspicion that this abnormality may exist, for example when the newborn can not keep milk down or 'chokes' constantly. To do this to every newborn can only be regarded as a very unpleasant welcome on this earth for the new little person.

If you want to actively help a baby who seems to struggle with amniotic fluid in its airway, you can use a nose sucker or your own mouth to help, but it is generally not necessary to do so.

... the placenta takes a long time to come out?

In hospital, but also at home, midwives are not keen to wait for the placenta a long time. Some time ago, we gave women 2 hours. But now, modern birth professional want to see a placenta within about 30 minutes after birth. At that point at the latest, but sometimes also earlier, they attempt to deliver the placenta by controlled cord traction – which can cause increased blood loss as well as discomfort and pain.

If the normal process of the third stage of labour is not interrupted, most placentas will be expelled within an hour of birth without much trouble. But there are cases where a placenta takes its time. Reports of placentas staying in place for one or more days after birth exist. This is rather rare however and should be regarded as the exception to the norm.

A placental phase of around 2 hours can be regarded as normal after an undisturbed birth. The gynaecologist and advocate for undisturbed birth Sven Hildebrandt considers 4 hours as the normal limit. (Hildebrandt 2008)

The most important thing to watch out for is increased blood loss that weakens the mother. A small amount of bleeding is normal and you can await a placenta that takes its time as long as there are no signs of a fever and therefore infection. But this can not be taken as absolute reassurance that all is well.

Squatting and gentle pulling on the cord by the mother herself while gently pushing some time after birth are generally sufficient to make the placenta appear, especially if the baby has already suckled at the breast. A famous German doctor, Willibald Pschyrembel (1901–1987) coined a famous phrase, nowadays mostly ignored due to easy access to operating theatres and blood transfusions: *'In the third stage of labour, the uterus is a temple. Hands off the uterus!'* (Pschyrembel 1947)

A delayed separation of the placenta from the uterine wall (and also heavy bleeding) can happen if the temperature of the water in the birthing pool is too high. A frequently overlooked reason for a delay is also the premature cutting and clamping of the umbilical cord before the placenta is delivered. Once the cord has stopped pulsing,

the baby does not need the placenta anymore but it seems the placenta receives signals from the baby to encourage separation from the uterine wall. (Hildebrandt 2008).

Many hospital transfers from home and freebirths for 'retained placentas' could be avoided if we had a little more patience. If a woman moves to the hospital from a freebirth because her placenta is still in situ, it generally turns out to be detached and sitting in the cervix, which makes it easy for birth professionals to remove it. The stress of transfer can be avoided in those cases. I have read about this exact scenario in several birth stories.

After a previous caesarean section, an (overly thorough) D&C or other procedures or operations involving the uterus, it is possible for the placenta to be abnormally strongly adhered to the scar tissue on the uterine wall and require professional help to separate. Forceful removal of the placenta in these cases specifically, both at home and in the hospital, can lead to a post partum haemorrhage.

Doctors are not agreed on the best procedure to deal with cases of abnormally adhered placentas. The procedure in most cases is a manual removal of the placenta from the uterus, but another school of thought is to see if nature will deal with the problem by itself. This is to minimise the risk of potentially life threatening blood loss that more frequently develops with traditional management and can cost the woman her uterus. In some places the placenta is even left in place as long as the mother does not lose too much blood.

Basically: Try to pass the placenta gently some time after birth under your own steam, or calmly wait a little bit longer and try again. As long as there is no heavy, continuous bleeding, there is no need to hurry and start interventions for the sake of speeding up the third stage by a few minutes and risk complications.

... I bleed heavily after the birth?

Gregory White (1921–2003) writes the following in his book 'Emergency Childbirth', and I quote as he summarises the most important issues beautifully:

'Luckily, women rarely die quickly from a post partum haemorrhage (PPH). The biggest blood loss after birth is generally fairly short lived and stops before it becomes a life threatening problem. A dangerous post partum haemorrhage is often a slow, continuous trickle. A new study examining 52 cases of women who died from PPH (without medical help – added by author) showed that none of these women died in the first 1.5 hours after birth. This means that helpers nearly always have time to seek medical help.'

Stories like: 'I lost x litres of blood and I had to be operated on straight away or I would have died.' are common. But we have to remember that births in hospital are often heavily interfered with. Be it episiotomies, purple pushing, suboptimal birthing positions or rough tugging of the umbilical cord, these interventions are not without consequence.

Routine induction and augmentation of labour increase the risk of haemorrhage due to the interruption of the normal hormonal interplay during birth. Even birth on your back can lead to heavy bleeding if the vena cava was (partially) occluded ('vena cava syndrome').

The body automatically reacts with a dilatation of the maternal blood vessels to compensate. Most women feel sick if this happens. Most pregnant women are already familiar with this from pregnancy: They can only lie on their backs for a short amount of time. This can persist for some time after birth.

To prevent an excessive bleed after a long and exhausting birth, potentially caused by a lack of calcium in your body's cells, prophylactic supplementation with **calcium** has proven helpful (perhaps with water soluble tablets). This can be drunk in sips as soon as contractions get weaker (as sign that calcium is lacking). Drinking plenty of fluids can also prevent heavy bleeding.

If the birth goes well and you are well nourished, life threatening bleeds are rare.

If a **haemorrhage** occurs after birth, there are several things that can help the uterus to contract and therefore stop it:

- **Put the baby to the breast.** The baby's suckling makes you produce oxytocin which in turn makes the uterus contract.

- **Place a small piece of placenta under your tongue.** This might sound brutal, but anecdotally, the effect is often instant. The placenta seems to contain a high concentration of hormones that tell your body: the baby is out, you can close the floodgates.

- **Put a bag of ice on your belly.** The cold stimulates the uterus to contract.

- **Massage your uterus so it contracts and squeeze it so it can't fill up with blood.** All the blood that accumulates in the uterus is taken from the mother's circulatory system.

- **Syntocinon** is routinely given in hospitals to speed up the birth of the placenta. The recommended dose differs in literature and is primarily based on anecdotal evidence. The manufacturers recommend 5–10 international units intramuscularly or 5–6 units slowly intravenously as treatment for uterine atonic bleeding, which is a bleed due to a relaxed uterus. (Rath 2008)

It is also possible to administer syntocinon drops or spray either nasally or bucally (through the oral mucous membranes).

Oxytocin used to be sold in Germany to support milk production but has been taken off the market as studies to support its use for this purpose were lacking.

You can still order oxytocin spray over the internet though and keep it, just in case it should become necessary to deal with a PPH. Make sure you are able to give a large enough dose with spray or drops, amounting to about 10 international units.

- **Massage:** Gently massage your uterus through the skin of your belly. The mother herself can do this as well as a helper. When the uterus reacts to this with a contraction it will feel firm and the bleeding should stop.

After massage, stay on your side for at least five minutes while squeezing the uterus tight with both hands.

As your abdomen will feel soft and stretched right after birth and the uterus is still fairly large, you should be able to pull it forward and kink it slightly with one hand behind it and the other in front. This is to ensure that the bleeding does not start up again. (White 1998)

A helper can be life saving in certain situations when the mother is unable to compress the uterus herself.

The uterus is essentially a vessel that needs to be held together to stop persistent bleeding if it can't do it by itself after birth.

There are also **specific herbs** which can be used to stem bleeding. Particularly effective are:

- **Angelica (angelica archangelica):** as a tea or tincture. This herb is said to stimulate the uterus and facilitate the delivery of placenta, as well as ease menstrual problems (Clark 2004). You should start with small doses as some people react strongly to its active ingredients.

- **Shepherd's Purse (capsella bursapastoris):** as tea or tincture. Said to reduce bleeding generally or after birth. Some authors consider this herb just as valuable as syntocinon (McLean 1998)

- **Motherwort:** also regarded as a uterine stimulant helpful after birth (Lin JH 2009)

Another thing: Talk to your uterus! Tell it what you need it to do. That sounds silly perhaps, but: body and soul are closely connected and influence each other. And you can use this connection to your advantage.

The following questions often come up in the context of postnatal blood loss:

- How do I know how much blood I have lost?

- And how can I tell when the loss becomes problematic?

A tip to answer the first question: You can check out what a half a litre or a litre of blood might look like either on a tarpaulin or perhaps the bath (in the case of a waterbirth). No one needs to donate blood for this, diluted ketchup or water with food dye and flour mixed to the right consistency will also do.

A blood loss larger than 500mls is classed as a post partum haemorrhage (a larger loss than normal).

One study comes to the conclusion that a loss over 1000mls should be treated as a PPH (Jouppila 1995).

The main problem is that even the professionals have problems estimating the exact amount of blood lost. Estimating the amount visually is so inaccurate, that it is nearly of no value to diagnose a PPH. (Schorn 2010)

A better way to estimate loss is weighing anything used to catch the blood before and after birth. The difference in grams approximately reflects the loss in millilitres. Another very important guide is the mother's condition. If she feels alert and can concentrate on her surroundings, the blood loss was likely not critical. The weaker and more tired she feels, the more significant the loss.

The following **emergency measures** are indicated after a large blood loss:

- if the bleeding continues after all the above measures have been taken, call an ambulance and continue to compress the uterus through the abdominal wall to keep blood loss as low as possible.

- if the bleeding has stopped, acute danger has passed. To hydrate and avoid shock, drink a litre of water with a teaspoon of salt and half a teaspoon of bicarbonate of soda dissolved in it (White 1989). Homemade bone or vegetable broth has a similar effect.

Typical symptoms of haemorrhage are tiredness, thirst, dizziness, problems with your circulation, whooshing noises in your ears, feeling cold, shaking, rapid pulse and, in severe cases loss of consciousness. Should the latter occur, a blood transfusion in the hospital may be indicated. The official treatment line for a blood transfusion in hospital is generally a haemoglobin level of 7–8 g/dl or below. (Pötsch 1997)

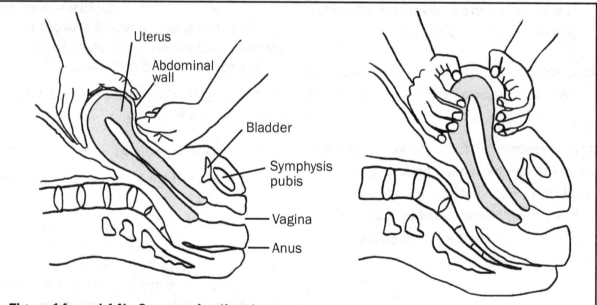

Figure 14a and 14b: Compressing the uterus
There are two methods to compress the uterus after birth to stop excessive bloodloss. You need to squeeze hard enough to stop the bleeding. Note in 14a, the fist is pushing the uterus back and upwards towards the spine, while the other hand is massaging the fundus to stimulate a contraction. Once the bleeding stops, use the method in 14b to keep the uterus compressed for a further 5 minutes.

Without a transfusion it is possible to compensate for blood loss with good nutritious, iron rich foods and appropriate supplements. Please expect it to take at least 6 weeks to raise haemoglobin to normal levels again.

A heavy bleed usually occurs only when the placenta has been detached from the uterus, as the vessels that previously connected the placenta and uterus are severed. For a few moments, after the placenta shears off the uterine wall, the vessels are not closed off and you see what is called a 'separation bleed'. If the mechanism that closes off those bleeding vessels fails, a haemorrhage occurs until the uterus finally does its 'job'.

In some cases, for example in the case of a malformation of the uterus, a heavy bleed occurs before the placenta is born without being caused by obstetric interference. In those cases the placenta needs to be born as quickly as possible.

If the above measures to stimulate the uterus do not work, a manual removal of placenta needs to be considered. This means inserting one hand into the uterus to scoop the placenta off the uterine wall.

A haemorrhage with a placenta still attached to the uterus is life threatening and requires immediate professional help, it is however a rare occurrence during an intervention free birth.

Even a placenta that has implanted very firmly into a uterine scar (from previous caesarean section or D&C) is usually delivered without problems, but small chunks of placenta can stay behind. Small chunks can be ignored initially as once the bulk of placenta has left the uterus, it can do its postnatal work and contract.

A slight but persistent bleed needs to be monitored carefully. It may not seem particularly dramatic initially, but can lead to an accumulative haemorrhage. Normally, blood will collect on the pad under the woman and clot to look like jelly. Once blood starts soaking into the pad without clotting, the clotting factors inherent in the blood may be running out.

If the bleed does not stop at that point it becomes life threatening for the mother. Feel your belly. The uterus should be palpable as a hard ball around belly button height. If it is higher up and soft, let your baby suckle at your breast and put a bag of ice (or a bag of frozen peas) wrapped in a kitchen towel on your belly.

If the uterus is firm, a slow steady bleed may well originate from a perineal or vaginal tear. Check your perineum and vagina with a hand mirror as thoroughly as possible. If you have sustained a large bleeding tear (which is rather unlikely during a freebirth) push a towel against the tear for about 15 minutes. If this does not help, it may be necessary to let someone suture the tear to stop the bleed.

Another reason for a long slow bleed may be retained pieces of placenta in the uterus. You can assume this is the case if there is no obvious trauma to vagina or perineum and the uterus feels doughy and does not appear to be contracting sufficiently.

Should you decide to take a watchful approach for now (regardless of where the blood is coming from) make sure you get up every few hours during the first night to go to the toilet. That way you can check if the bleeding has stopped or not. If you stay in bed all night, blood can pool in the vagina and you may only notice a critical loss when attempting to get up in the morning, at which point you may be close to circulatory collapse and might not be able to get up.

At this point and in the context of postnatal bleeding I would like to mention the 'active management of third stage' that has been routine in hospitals for the last 50 years. This management attempts to minimise the risks of excessive post-partum blood loss.

Common for this management is the administration of syntocinon and ergometrine, usually intramuscularly after the birth of the baby's anterior shoulder or the whole baby, the immediate clamping and cutting of the cord and controlled cord traction to deliver the placenta – not rarely unpleasant and painful for the mother.

All the components of the 'active management of third stage' methodology have been examined with regards to their efficiency to prevent PPH, and it has been concluded that only the administration of an oxytocic (such as syntocinon, a medication that helps the uterus contract) has a beneficial effect (Aflaifel 2012). As such, syntocinon can be useful to treat uterine atony. However, the routine prophylactic administration of oxytocics after every birth has not been proven to be beneficial. (Hildebrandt 2008)

If the mother has already received oxytocics to speed up the birth, she will need far larger amounts of this synthetic hormone to stop a postpartum bleed than women who have not. The mother's body develops a tolerance to the higher dose of oxytocics, thereby depressing its own production of oxytocin and becoming desensitised to further doses given. (Phaneuf 1997 & 2000)

Furthermore, large bleeds after birth occur more frequently in women who had an augmented labour as the artificially stimulated uterus tires more quickly and struggles to contract. (Balki 2013)

The best thing is to enable the mother to produce her own oxytocin (the natural form of syntocinon) from the start. And this is most likely to occur in a relaxed environment, such as her own home. This conclusion is supported by many freebirth stories that mostly report a surprisingly small amount of blood loss.

Birth and pain

The chances of a painless birth are greatest if it takes place in an undisturbed and self determined environment, in the protection of your own home or in another place of your choosing. Many internet videos show women birthing their babies easily and with joy.

As much as I would love birth to be like that for each and every woman: Most of them – even those who prepared with hypnobirthing, or other breathing and meditation techniques – are confronted with some pain and effort at the time of birth.

Regarding pain and birth, there are varying opinions in the home and freebirth 'scene'. Amongst those are the 'hardliners', who think pain has no place in birth and a woman who is truly relaxed and free of fear will feel no pain. Being that experience paints a somewhat different picture, I think the process of birth is likely more complex and can not be reduced to our thought processes and the power of our imagination only.

In my opinion, the physical condition also plays a role. The baby's position and size, the mother's pelvic shape and the ability to adapt to the enormous stretching of soft tissues need to be taken into account ...

At the end of the day it is the pain that encourages the woman to stay mobile and change her position and breathing. Pain can lead intuition to do the right thing.

We can influence many things, but not all. During birth we need an openness to accept that everything that happens makes sense.

I have so far given birth to four babies in an undisturbed and self-directed way. Two of those births were quick and essentially pain free. During the others, there was some pain involved, certainly in transition but also during the pushing phase. But it wasn't the kind of pain women describe when they are at the mercy of the process and helplessly beg for an epidural. However, at a certain point all my learned relaxation techniques failed me. Labour became so intense that I could not remain completely relaxed. Most birth stories report similar. This is the moment some German midwives describe as 'passing through the gates'.

So what should you do if the sensations of labour become so intense that the practiced relaxation techniques don't work anymore? First of all, realise that this is entirely normal. It is sometimes helpful to clarify in your own head which phase of labour you are dealing with. Most of the time you will find that you are in transition, and will shortly start getting the urge to push. It is nearly over and you can see light at the end of the tunnel.

And if it helps: scream, swear, laugh, make dirty jokes ... probably only elite athletes experience a similar intensity as we do in this moment.

If you find that you are not yet in transition, it might be worth having a think and a word with the baby as to why it might be that your labour is so painful. By listening closely to your body, you might find you instinctively know how to move to coax your baby into a better position.

To read more about help positioning the baby for birth, see page 85.

Protecting the perineum, episiotomy and perineal tears

Midwives learn how to protect your perineum when the head is being born. But they also learn to cut the perineum.

Probably due to invasive obstetrics and suboptimal birthing positions, the myth of uncontrollable ripping of the perineum came into existence. That is when someone thought it was probably better to cut the perineum prophylactically to outwit out of control nature. Moreover, it was thought that this would save women from incontinence and prolapse in later life.

So they got busy with the scissors – especially for first time mothers. These days, all the hypothetical reasons to perform an episiotomy have been disproven.

A cut does not prevent a tear (how could it possibly do that?) and it also does not protect from more severe perineal tearing. In fact, it makes more severe tearing, incorporating the anal muscles, more likely. Neither does it protect against incontinence or prolapse (Klein & Gauthier 1994, Hartmann & Viswanathan 2005, de Tayrac 2006). But there are still many (old school) midwives who cut perineums.

We can protect ourselves against overeager midwives performing episiotomies by not consenting to the use of episiotomy scissors or by birthing alone. As already mentioned in the previous information about perineal massage, the perineum does not require special preparation to be ready for birth. The hormones present in the perineal tissues and other parts of the body during birth enable you to stretch as much as necessary without sustaining (significant) injuries.

If a woman is able to move instinctively during a freebirth, no further explanation is necessary. You will do what you need to do to protect your perineum adequately. Sounds presumptuous? Never mind.

Of course there is still the part of our brain that wants to rationalise and understand everything in advance. We have been taught that life goes on only if we power ahead with a brain working overtime and incredible strength of will.

This is why I will give you some pointers that you will find out for yourself anyway, just before your baby's head is born:

- **Be upright,** this makes sure the pressure of the head on the perineum is as even as possible. Many women choose to be on all fours.

- **Only push** when you feel you need to.

- **Touch your perineum** and feel the head if you wish to. Some women like a warm compress on their perineum if they are not already in water.

- **Open your mouth,** let your jaw go slack and moan, lustily, as if in pain or both. It doesn't matter how. The main thing is to relax your mouth up top as this means your cervix and pelvic floor down low are also relaxed.

- **You will feel the urge to push** and a curiously urgent burning sensation, when the head is in your vagina. Perhaps you will slow down your pushing consciously and breathe especially deeply so you don't stretch too fast. Admittedly, some women cannot resist the enormous urge to push at this point and push with almighty force. Generally the damage from this superfast stretch is limited to harmless grazes and will heal by itself.

Once you have welcomed your baby and birthed the placenta, sooner or later you will likely feel the need to freshen up. There will be some blood (and possibly other bodily emissions) stuck to your legs and you are probably curious to know if your perineum is intact.

> If you don't feel any burning when you urinate, it is likely that you don't have any significant injuries to your perineum. Take a small mirror into the shower and check your perineum to be certain.

You hopefully already know what your vagina normally looks like, so it should be easy to see if something does not look like it should.

Here is some information about how birth can change your vagina:

There are **perineal tears**, **vaginal wall tears** and **grazes**. Perineal tears are divided into 4 grades, grade 3 and 4 (tears incorporating the anal sphincter and potentially rectal mucosa) are rare in births free of rough intervention. Grade 1 and 2 describe superficial and deep tearing of the back of the vagina.

If the perineal muscles are severed during a tear, they should be sutured to maintain their function during sexual intercourse. Small tears generally heal without long term issues and aesthetic concerns.

You can also have tears treated at home by your partner. For smaller tears that do sometimes happen even during freebirths, you can use special glue for wounds (Ezra 2014). The active ingredient in special glue for wounds (2-octyl cyanoacrylate) is nearly identical to the ingredient in super glue (cyanoacrylate) so the latter can theoretically be used for wounds as well, as it was before special wound glue was invented. 2-octyl cyanoacrylate was invented especially to be more gentle and elastic for its intended purpose. (Greene 1999)

Grazes are generally superficial and don't require any special treatment.

For any tearing, it is recommended to only open your legs as far as absolutely necessary (for example to go to the toilet) so as to avoid interrupting the healing process.

> If you feel – after awaiting events initially – that your tear needs some stitches, you might be best served by an experienced midwife willing to come to your home. However this should happen within the first 24 hours as after this time, the healing process is too far advanced for efficient repair.

For completeness sake I would like to mention that tight suturing with too many stitches can lead to problems. This is why a continuous suturing method (figure of eight technique by Rockel-Loenhoff) is preferable if in any doubt. (Rockel-Loenhoff 2012)

Here is my story: During my first birth I sustained a vaginal tear that bled rather heavily due to coached pushing. My midwife was very experienced in suturing tears, but it is not always clear how things used to fit together before the tear (especially if there are small remnants of the vaginal hymen). Let's just say, my vagina looked somewhat different after that birth.

I was lucky and didn't suffer any problems from this tear or the stitches, but it did partially reopen during the next birth. I let this tear heal without any stitches and look much like I did before my first birth again.

It seems logical that the edges of a tear would easily fit together if you leave them alone, but if they are sewn together in a crooked fashion they will heal that way. These days I have lost all fear of tearing and know that my body is very good at repairing itself, should something break.

An injury to the anal sphincter is almost unheard of during freebirths as already mentioned and everything else – perhaps apart from a (rare) complete severing of the perineal muscles – normally heals by itself. At least that is my opinion. But of course I would not keep anyone from getting sutures if they feel they need them.

Suturing perineal or vaginal injuries can however make sense if they bleed a lot. Again, this is only to mention every possibility. I have yet to encounter such a case in all the freebirth stories I have read. More about how to find out where exactly the blood you are losing is coming from can be found on page 97.

Scar tissue from previous births, as far as I can tell from what affected women have told me, does not tend to present a problem. So despite extensive scar tissue you can expect to remain (mostly) intact during a subsequent birth.

Cutting the cord – how, when and what with?

'And what did you do with the cord?'

This is the most frequent question I get asked when I tell people about our way of birth. Usually it is uttered with a mix of wonder and astonishment. When I simply answer: 'We just cut it.'

A disbelieving stare usually follows and then the realisation that explains everything to them about our masterful performance: 'Yeah well, I guess you are doctors.'

This, I find really irritating. I have never seen the simple act of cutting my baby's cord in the context of my medical qualifications. Everyone who has scissors and the motoric ability to work them, can cut a cord. What is so complicated about this process that people think you require a hospital or a medically qualified person to do it?

Looking at the animal kingdom you will find pretty careless treatment of umbilical cords. Once I observed the birth of a calf and the cord simply snapped as the mother cow stood up to lick her newborn clean. One end just dangled from where the calf had just emerged from. The other end (with hardly any length to it) was a bloody stump on the calf lying in the straw enjoying the vigorous licking by its mother.

Cord clamp? Sterile scissors? No. Mama cow and her offspring did not seem bothered by this and the calf survived as far as I know.

Realistically it happens all the time. All creatures who are equipped with an umbilical cord in their mothers' bellies manage without professional cutting of the cord at birth. No one calls for a doctor or a cord clamp. More likely is that things happen rather roughly: it gets either chewed off, bitten off or simply rips off. Just as long as it's off.......but definitely not sterile.

Why do we humans make things so complicated? Do we need professionals and rituals to see the survival of our offspring as guaranteed? When I say: 'We just cut it.' I often have the feeling people don't actually believe me. But we did just that. When we'd welcomed the new baby for long enough, the cord had long stopped pulsing and placenta was out. So out came the kitchen scissors and the cord was cut.

Admittedly: after our first birth alone, my husband felt more comfortable tying a thread around the baby's end of the cord, despite me waiting for half a day to cut the cord at all. The placenta had long since been expelled. But once you have started questioning societal norms and fears and decide to think for yourself, you thankfully soon forget the need for fear eliminating rituals.

Instead you learn that the umbilical cord is an amazing thing: it not only nourished your baby for its nine months in utero, it also knows how to stick together internally and cease its function when it is not needed after birth.

A few minutes after birth, the cord generally stops the blood flow and the walls of its vessels collapse. There might be a few blood clots here and there, and the inside of the cord is still moist which is why the cord stump tends to keep oozing fluid and tiny amounts of blood (you can always tie it off if you would like to avoid that) – but this is only blood not required by the baby anymore.

So why is there so much fear surrounding the severing of the cord? Do we believe the baby could suddenly start bleeding heavily through the cord stump and exsanguinate? Or are we afraid of bacteria making the baby ill?

If you have fears like that or similar ones, you may feel calmer if you use a cord tie or perhaps a sterile cord clamp – like in the hospital – and wait a few hours before actually cutting the cord. You can also leave an extra long stump of cord (and trim it down later).

I recently read an article about newborn tetanus in some third world countries. It is very common there to use cow dung in their care for the cord stump. Well, something as stupid as that will of course have consequences, or so we may think.

However, with a little more background knowledge, a whole different picture appears:

Cow dung application has been traditional cord care forever. The cases of tetanus infection only started rising when midwives trained in a western way of birth started trimming cords very close to the baby's umbilicus. Until then, traditionally, cords used to be cut close to the placenta. What sort of bacteria would go such a long way through a stuck together cord? This is where traditional and western practices mix in a harmful way. But instead of recognising this, we insist on even more western practices: tetanus vaccination will surely sort it out.

So is it true that only a professional in a hospital can safely cut an umbilical cord? No, unless you want to cut the cord immediately after birth before it has ceased pulsing and is empty of blood as is commonly done in hospitals (to check cord blood for pH levels and for quality control). If you do that, then the cord does indeed have a lot of blood flowing through it still and you would need all the medical paraphernalia to avoid a blood bath.

 You might want to go down a different route and do nothing at all. This is called 'lotus birth'. You take care of the placenta until the umbilical stump heals and falls off together with its placenta.

Another word about cord blood and timing of cord cutting: in hospital you can donate your baby's cord blood to treat other sick children. There are also firms which freeze the harvested cord blood for a fee in case your baby gets sick at some point and might benefit from the stem cells in its cord blood at a later date.

In reality this might be wasting your money. If stem cell therapy becomes necessary for your child, it does not make sense to use stem cells with the same genetic problem as your child's.

What if a sibling or other family member becomes sick? Of course then stem cells with the same or similar genetic material may well be helpful. You have to ask yourself if you feel it is important to prepare for this unlikely scenario or not.

To donate cord blood, but also without this reason, staff in hospitals often cut cords before they have stopped pulsing and sometimes collect the cord blood. Studies show that it is far better to wait until the pulsing has stopped so that the baby receives all the precious stem cells within the cord blood itself.

Early cord clamping (a minute after birth) potentially robs the baby of approximately 30–40% of its blood volume and 60% of its red blood cells. Babies whose cords are cut later (more than a minute after birth or after pulsing of the cord has stopped) have measurably higher haemoglobin levels and are less likely to suffer from anaemia between three and six months old. (McDonald 2013)

During a freebirth, no one ever has the idea to cut the cord before it has stopped pulsing. If you have to birth your baby in the hospital, you need to tell your caregivers firmly that you would like to wait to cut the cord until it has stopped pulsing, even better, until the placenta has been expelled, or that you want it to stay intact altogether for a lotus birth.

In connection with the cutting of the cord, professionals often insist that the baby needs to be below or at uterus height so that the blood from the baby does not flow back into the placenta, leaving the baby with too little blood. This is only true for a lifeless baby without blood pressure. The system 'baby-placenta' is designed in such a way that it enables the baby to get all the blood it requires and that its pulmonary circulation works without a hitch as long as you leave the cord intact.

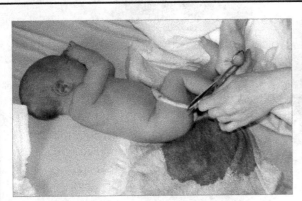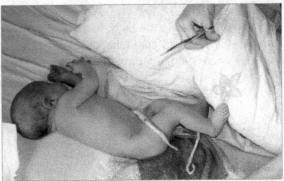

Cutting the cord with normal scissors – in this case 12 hours after birth. The placenta is wrapped in a towel. A spontaneous, not very effective solution as fluid is draining from the placenta. With the next baby we unromantically used a practical plastic bag. With the last baby we didn't wait as long to cut the cord and didn't need a special receptacle for the placenta. During a planned lotus birth the placenta is usually kept in a bowl or a special placenta pouch until the cord drops off by itself.

Checking the placenta

The placenta is a soft, flat organ that is similar to raw liver or pancake (from the latin placenta = cake) in consistency and appearance. To take a closer look, put it on a large flat plate.

The first thing you will notice is that the placenta has two different sides. The smooth side faces the baby during pregnancy and has the cord attached to its middle. You can see any vessels running towards the cord's attachment in the centre, forming a starlike pattern.

The opposite side was attached to the uterine wall. It looks like a gently hilly landscape or even like the surface of a cauliflower. White hard dots are calcifications that can occur towards the end of pregnancy.

The side that was attached needs to be checked for completeness. If single hills or parts of hills are missing and parts of the surface seem like they have chunks pulled out, it is likely there are placental leftovers in the uterus still. Generally though, after a normal, pain free placenta delivery, the placenta is complete. Should this not be the case and to learn how to spot this, see page 134 for the subject of lochia.

The membranes that surrounded the baby in utero are attached to the margin of the placenta. If you spread them out with your fingers, it is easy to imagine how they contained the baby. You can also see the tear in the amniotic sac that released the baby.

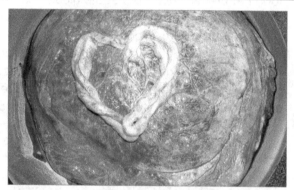

This is the side facing the baby. In the middle you can see the attached cord (shaped into a heart), note part of the membranes on the margin.

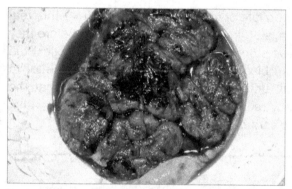

Typical structure of the opposite side of the placenta, membranes visible surrounding it.

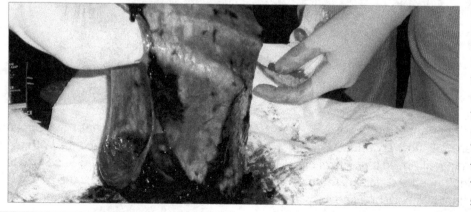

After birth, check that the placenta is complete. A midwife can do this (as on this occasion, hence the gloves) or you can do it yourself. The baby exited the amniotic sac through the tear shown.

So now you have a baby and a placenta. What to do with the baby is mostly obvious. But what do you do with the placenta?

- You can simply and unromantically **put it in the rubbish bin** (much frowned upon in the UK as it can lead to a search for an abandoned newborn if discovered, however unlikely this may be)

- A fairly well known tradition is to **bury** the placenta and plant a tree on top of it.

- Some like to make a placenta **smoothie** with a piece of the placenta. You can design it to your own liking.

  Here is a sample recipe:

  1 piece of placenta (approximately 8cm in diameter)
  1 banana
  2 handfuls of berries
  50–150mls water
  And blend.

Raw placenta is said to help the uterus shrink back down to pre pregnancy size and increase milk production. To achieve the same thing you can also have a homeopathic remedy made from your placenta. Placentas disposed of in hospital often end up in the cosmetic industry.

If you are not quite sure what to do with your placenta, you can always freeze it for the time being. For more creative suggestions regarding the placenta, there are some books on the market you can check out.

Freebirth under difficult circumstances

When you don't have any support

Many women manage to convince their other halves that a freebirth is the best thing for them.

However, some men can not be convinced of such plans despite extensive efforts. Not even if you promise the attendance of a midwife. The last thing you need in labour is a partner who is afraid and calls the ambulance as soon as something seems 'dangerous' to him.

In the case of an anxious partner, you have three options:

- You do what your partner wants and go to hospital to have your baby

- You come to a compromise. Find a solution agreeable for both of you by changing your preferences a little bit. The outcome depends on your bargaining skills.

- If your partner does not support you, do your own thing anyway.

I have read women's stories who kept labour a secret until it was too late to go anywhere, an ambulance could not be called in time or who managed to send their partners on a lovely trip into town or on a day trip with friends etc.

Another problem can be a husband being in full agreement but other family members being difficult. Not only verbally but in a very creative and aggressive manner.

Reports to police about a husband keeping his wife from going to the hospital have happened. As have visits from social services and police.

Couples have left their homes and taken up residence in hotels or elsewhere to escape from well meaning family and have their babies in peace.

These stories show that you need to be careful who you tell of your freebirth plans. Sometimes it is better to be vague and only go into details after the event.

Even then it can be difficult to calm down shocked friends and family.

Freebirth and breech presentation

3 to 5% of babies present by the breech with their feet or bottom at the time of labour. The closer the labour to the EDB, the lower the likelihood the baby will be born breech.

In the year 2000, a large, but very questionable study showed that a caesarean section may be safer for a baby presenting by the breech than a vaginal birth (Hannah 2000). The caesarean section rate for breech babies rose dramatically following this and hardly any babies presenting by the breech are born vaginally these days. The study was met with much criticism regarding methodology and study design and a retraction was even requested. (Glezerman 2006)

Later studies found that vaginal birth under good conditions leads to the same outcomes for breech babies as a birth by caesarean section (Alarab 2004, Goffinet 2006). In some places, this led to a rethink for many birth professionals, but there is still much debate about the optimal route of birth due to the lack of practical experience. If there are statistically significant differences between vaginal and caesarean birth for those babies, they are very small indeed.

The maternal side of this debate, for example the problems a caesarean birth can cause with regards to future births and the fact the mother can certainly not be regarded as healthy after major abdominal surgery, is generally disregarded in studies such as these. Another thing ignored is that most of the studied births happened with the mother on her back which makes birthing, particularly a breech baby, more difficult in itself.

Breech babies generally require more time to transition from intrauterine life to an extrauterine one than their little head down friends. Also, the mortality rate for breech babies seems around 2–4% higher than for cephalic babies, regardless of mode of birth (caesarean vs vaginal) (Fischer 2012). This difference is diminished if you take out complications caused by prematurity (which is often correlated with a birth in breech presentation). (Weiss 1998)

It follows that a caesarean for breech presentation does not save lives but is primarily carried out due to birth professionals' inexperience, convenience and fear.

Relevant physical anomalies (fibroids of the uterus, malformation of the uterus) or skeletal problems (issues with spine or pelvis) as well as awkward placental positioning (low lying placenta or placenta praevia) play a rather small role in persistent breech presentation.

Some babies are slow to turn head down because their 'righting reflex' is yet to be developed (perhaps due to placental insufficiency). In a premature baby, this reflex has not developed yet either.

Also, women who have had several babies are more likely to have breech babies (Fischer 2012). Moreover, a tense pelvic floor is a possible cause. Many women report that their baby turned after an osteopath treated their pelvis. In many cases, though, it is impossible to find a reason for the baby's refusal to move head down.

There are many tricks to encourage a baby to turn head down, for example the 'Indian bridge, 'shining the way' with a torch, acupuncture and moxibustion. More ways to coax your baby's head down are featured on page 61.

An 'external cephalic version' is only performed in hospitals with access to an operating theatre as the vigorous attempts at turning the baby from the outside carry the risk of placental abruption. This procedure is often not successful however and the baby might quickly turn back even if it was.

This shows clearly that this issue is not simply a mechanical one but a much more complex matter. Really, women who have a breech baby on board should not have to worry about their baby's birth. The vast majority of all babies will turn before labour starts and even during labour in some cases. And if not, it is mostly an issue for the inexperienced birth attendant rather than for the mother and her baby.

Because theoretically babies are 'deliverable' in any position, bar transverse and oblique lie.

The catchphrase for breech birth is: 'Hands off the breech!' This means that pulling or other forms of manipulation should be avoided, though one or two gently supporting hands are permissible.

Breech birth should take place in an upright position (standing, kneeling, on a birth stool or on all fours), utilising gravity without someone creating unnecessary problems by 'helping'. The baby will fold its arms and legs so that the body can pass the pelvis optimally. As long as the birth is progressing, experienced birth professionals will only make sure that the carefully formed tangle of baby does not 'unravel' before birth. Gravity usually ensures that the baby is born in a nicely tucked in fashion, so that outside handling to help, possibly apart from the gently supporting hand, does not become necessary.

The perineum does not need a (helper's) hand protecting it either. Breech babies are quite gentle on the perineum as the baby's bottom is much softer than the baby's head normally coming first.

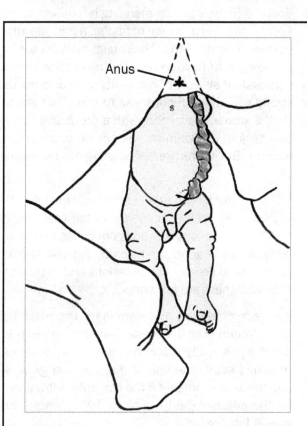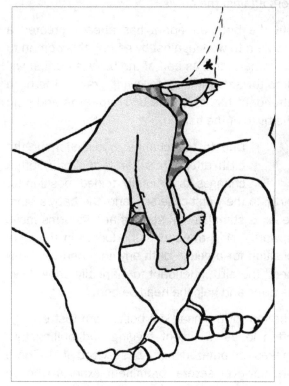

Figures 15a and 15b: Breech presentation birth
This is what a birth by the breech can look like. The mother is in a kneeling position while the baby's legs, rump, arms and last but not least the head are born. As a rule, no outside help is necessary for a breech birth if the mother is undisturbed and follows her baby's and her body's impulses.

However, what normally happens during breech births in hospital is this: the woman is put on her back. This often happens to make CTG monitoring easier and to facilitate vaginal examinations but during a breech birth, which is automatically classed as high risk, it becomes even more important it seems.

Fear is in the air and usually birth attendants are very much aware that they have less experience of this type of birth than ideally necessary. So intervention is used readily because it is believed that it might help avert danger.

As soon as bottom or feet are born, the birth attendant wants to achieve a quick birth of the head. The big fear is usually that the baby's blood supply will be cut off by the head compressing the cord against the pelvis.

But the birth attendant has already created a problem to work against by getting the woman to lie on her back. As half of the body is born, it will drop towards the bed, following gravity. The birth attendant has to lift the body upwards and help the birth of the head.

Due to the change in direction or the birth attendant's hands the baby often changes its optimally 'folded' position for birth. In the worst case scenario, the baby's Moro reflex is stimulated, it startles and its arms move upwards. Now the baby is no longer in the ideal position for a gentle birth anymore and will likely need the birth attendant to manually bring down its arms and help the head be born.

The fear of the head not being born fast enough often leads to violent tugging and pulling that makes you amazed the baby survived at all. There are however several prominent experts who do not feel that the baby's cord gets so compressed during a breech birth that it presents a danger. (Rockenschaub 2005)

Luckily on the internet you can find amazing videos, alongside not so positive ones, that show breech birth as positive and physically gentle for women with the help of calm and reserved birth attendants. (Barrett 2008)

So: don't fear a breech birth, but be wary of unskilled and fearful birth attendants. And think about this: No one has forced your baby into a breech presentation. Trust that your baby is able to withstand the consequences of its freely chosen birth presentation. Our children do many things that we do not regard as ideal, but they usually find their own solutions anyway.

Freebirth after caesarean section

A woman who has already had one or more children via caesarean section often encounters particular difficulties while planning her dream birth. Apart from the challenge of finding a midwife supportive of homebirth in these circumstances, she will likely also have to face the resistance of the established system of maternity care and needs strong will and stubbornness to reach her goals. On the whole, the mother with a previous section can be just as optimistic as any other pregnant woman. But there are a few things to be aware of:

After a caesarean section you are left with a scar on your uterus. In the vast majority of cases this does not cause any problems during a subsequent birth, but you should know how to prevent complications and to be able to react if there are any concerns.

It is recommended to determine if the placenta is implanted over the caesarean scar and to rule out the possibility that it has grown into it via ultrasound scan. The risk of the placenta growing into the scar is present if the placenta is low down on the anterior uterine wall, which is where the scar is located.

If the placenta is implanted elsewhere, you do not have to worry about this issue. And if the placenta is sitting over the scar, do not worry unduly. Should there be problems with the separation of the placenta, the same course of action as described in 'What if ... the placenta takes a long time to come out?' on page 92 can be taken.

There is also the small possibility of the scar on the uterine wall reopening during pregnancy or birth. In the worst case scenario, the baby can exit the uterus through the hole in the scar and end up in the abdominal cavity where it is cut off from its oxygen supply if the placenta detaches from the uterus. The risk of scar rupture, depending on study, is approximately 0.3–0.6%. (Chauhan 2003, Spong 2007)

The number of previous caesarean sections does not seem to influence the rate of ruptures significantly, however the risk of a placenta being abnormally adherent to the uterine scar or a placenta praevia does rise with each section performed. (Silver 2006)

The likelihood of rupture also rises if there were any difficulties with wound healing or fever after the previous section. However, each vaginal birth after previous caesarean section lowers the risk of scar rupture. (Mercer et al 2008)

Not all caesarean section scars are equal. Generally, a caesarean incision is made horizontally in the lower third of the uterus. This type of scar has the lowest risk of rupture. A significantly higher risk of rupture is attached to a scar in the upper part of the uterus or a vertical incision. This type of incision may have been used during breech caesareans, premature births, uterine malformations or under extremely emergent circumstances.

Which type of incision you have had is not immediately noticeable as the outer scar on the skin does not necessarily correspond to the scar on your uterus. If in doubt and to get a clear picture, request a viewing of your notes.

To keep the strain on your scar and therefore the rupture risk low, the following points are important:

- **Strive for a gentle birth without induction.** Studies show that inductions (for example with prostaglandins) increase the risk of scar rupture significantly. (Kayani 2005) Even inductions with other uterine stimulants as well as castor oil should be avoided.

- **Change your nutrition and potentially reduce your weight** in case of obesity, if possible even before pregnancy.

- **Leave a sufficient gap before having your next baby** after caesarean section. The gap should ideally be at least two years.

Measuring the thickness of your uterine scar by ultrasound only has very little predictiveness with regards to your risk factors. It certainly should not be the sole deciding factor for your plans.

The question of how you could possibly plan to have a homebirth or even freebirth with a history of one or more caesarean sections comes up again and again. Is it not extremely dangerous?

As always, every woman has to weigh up her risk factors individually for herself and her situation. For me personally, a calm birth at home would have been extremely important for me after a lower segment caesarean section, despite the low but undeniable risk of rupture.

In hospital, vaginal births after caesarean (VBAC) are often induced or augmented without regard for the previous history, although we know that this increases the risk of rupture. It is also very common to switch off the woman's sensations with an epidural.

However, the woman's feeling that something is not as it should be during contractions and between contractions is of great importance as a means to decide a plan of care. And generally, at home you have a bigger chance of a swift, uncomplicated labour which is gentle on the uterine scar.

For a woman who has only ever experienced a birth via caesarean section, it is likely reassuring to have an experienced midwife in the background who can help guide her through the emotionally and physically turbulent transition and to decide if potential pain is normal or indicative of problems with the scar.

The first signs of a scar about to rupture are stabbing, severe or niggling pains even in the break between contractions or even contractions weakening in general. If the scar has already ruptured, it is possible for the head to come back out of the pelvis and be felt above your symphysis pubis. An abnormal fetal heartbeat, lasting feelings of fear and worry in the mother, a subjective inkling that something is not quite right, tachycardia (fast heartbeat in the mother) and dropping blood pressure are all serious warning signals.

There are not many birth stories reporting a scar rupture as this event is thankfully very rare. Whoever wants to read more can however find some information on the internet and see how women experienced this emergency. A recurring issue seems to be that women were not immediately taken seriously with their concerns by hospital staff.

More often though you will find encouraging success stories of home and freebirths after one or more caesareans.

If you have to go to hospital

Do you have a medical issue that is likely to make birth more complicated for you and/or makes medical help necessary? Did you have serious problems in pregnancy or is it suspected that your newborn will require immediate medical attention?

If so, it might be possible that hospital is the best place of birth for you. You have to make this decision for yourself – hopefully informed and with the support of your partner – as it is you, who ultimately has to birth your baby. Your decision will depend on your individual situation, as well as your level of support and gut feeling.

You may also choose a hospital birth if you are unable to gain your partner's support.

A hospital birth can generally not be compared with one in the relaxed, undisturbed environment of home – that should be clear. But what is possible in hospitals varies widely, depending on how flexible the birth attendants are in accommodating the woman's wishes.

It is best to check in advance what specific hospitals are willing to do to accommodate those wishes and what sort of thing would be non negotiable.

Routines common in hospitals are CTG monitoring and regular vaginal examinations. It is also common to put in venous access (venflon) to be able to give drugs if necessary, such as labour augmenting drugs, often without much information.

There are guidelines regarding progress and length of labour. Episiotomies are not rare, neither is coached pushing. And still most hospital births happen with the woman on her back or in a semi sitting position.

However, there are some hospitals (some anthroposophical) which are very happy to respect the woman's individual wishes and forget about routines. To find out which hospital may be for you, you can ask the questions listed on the following page.

Furthermore, you should always check consent forms before signing them so you know exactly what you are consenting to.

Hospital staff are only authorised to do what they have consent for, so it makes sense to write down some birth preferences (also called a birth plan by some) to outline how you would like your birth to go, what you absolutely do not consent to and what you may consent to in certain circumstances.

An extensive list of such preferences can help you achieve your dream birth and good midwives will respect your wishes wherever possible.

Questions to ask before a planned hospital birth

Birth:

How many birthing rooms/birthing pools are available? How often do they get used?

How many midwives are on duty?

Can I bring my 'own' midwife?

How many doctors are on duty/on call?

Do you do Domino births?

Can I choose how many supporters I wish to have at my birth?

Is it possible to be alone for the birth/not be touched during birth?

What is your protocol for prelabour rupture of membranes? What are your time limits for intervention (induction/antibiotics)?

What are your protocols regarding VBAC or breech birth? What limitations do you put on women during such birth?

Do you use complementary medicine (acupuncture/homeopathy)?

Can I move around as I wish? How do you restrict movement?

Can I choose my own birthing position? Can I catch my own baby?

Am I allowed to eat and drink freely?

Is it possible to listen to my own music (are CD players available)?

What are your routine interventions? Episiotomy? Venflon? Artificial rupture of membranes? Continuous monitoring? (If so, on the bed, or do you have portable units?)

Is it possible to avoid a CTG? Can you listen to the baby's heart with a pinard?

How long are you happy to wait for the placenta before intervention is used to get it out?

When do you generally clamp and cut the cord? Can it wait until the placenta is delivered?

Do you suction newborns routinely? Do you suction their stomachs?

Do you only administer medications after birth (Vitamin K/eyedrops) if parents have consented?

Statistics:

How many women birth their baby upright rather than on their backs or semi sitting?

How many births happen with an epidural?

How many waterbirths do you have?

How many episiotomies do you perform?

How many labours are induced?

How many days post due dates do you wait until induction?

What is your caesarean section rate?

How many caesarean sections happen under general anaesthetic?

How many births happen via ventouse or forceps?

Questions regarding postnatal care:

Can I be discharged a couple of hours after birth?

Do you separate mother and baby at any time? Does the baby stay with me all the time?

Do I decide how long the baby stays with me after birth?

Can I breastfeed right after birth?

Do you support breastfeeding on demand (no feeding routine)?

Do you give dummies to newborns?

Do you top babies up with formula (only if there is a medical reason and the baby requires it)?

Do you seek consent from the parents with regards to giving formula supplements?

Do you use bottles to give supplements or alternative means (such as cup or spoon)?

Are there breastfeeding counsellors available or specially trained midwives?

Is there a separate breastfeeding room?

Can I limit the amount of visitors?

How many women per room? Are there single rooms/family rooms available so the father can also stay over?

In case the baby needs special care:

Is there a children's ward/neonatal intensive care unit?

Do you offer hip ultrasounds or hearing tests?

How often do babies get transferred to other hospitals?

If the baby does need transfer, where will it go?

I have however also read about birth plans being ignored completely – even in the most sympathetic hospitals. So consider the possibility that you may have lots of reassurance in the run up to labour but may be met with resistance and need to fight for what you want once you turn up in labour.

It is also advisable to mention in the birth preferences who will be your advocate when you are unable to (fully) decide for yourself when you are in labour. Your partner or a friend will be able to take the role or advocate and discuss matters with hospital staff so you don't have to concentrate on that when you are busy birthing your baby.

If you decide on a hospital birth it may be helpful to find a midwife who is willing and able to do a domino birth for you (conduct your antenatal care at home and accompany you to hospital for the birth) so you know who will attend the birth and don't have to worry about shift changes (although some mums find a change of midwife positive). An independent midwife can offer similar service.

Midwives offering this service however still have certain protocols, limitations, days off sick and holidays, so an unhindered birth in hospital is rare, but not impossible.

In the USA a woman named Lia Joy Rundle went into hospital to have her 4th baby after 3 free-births. After a turbulent pregnancy during which one twin died, she felt that it was the sensible thing to do. She birthed her baby in the bath tub despite waterbirth not officially being allowed in this particular hospital. She did have a midwife with her who was happy to respect her wishes and did not adhere to hospital protocol. By the way, her birth was completely uncomplicated despite fears to the contrary and can be viewed on YouTube ('The self-directed hospital birth of Zena Joy').

Water can be a great tool to achieve relaxation and privacy in a strange environment. Vaginal examinations and other interventions are less likely when you are in the water, simply because it makes it more uncomfortable for birth attendants to perform them.

Many hospitals have a birth pool women are at least allowed to labour in. Just before birth, women are coaxed out onto dry land, though some hospitals offer water birth as well. In reality though, many midwives still try to get women to get back on the bed just before birth. Some women just ignore this and stay in the pool anyway until the baby is born.

A means to escape continuous CTG monitoring is the toilet. If necessary, you simply need the toilet very frequently and stay as long as possible, shielded from view and able to stay upright and mobile. Lock the door if you want.

And of course, the 'classic' tip: Whatever you do, don't go to the hospital too soon. Labour often slows dramatically or stops altogether with a change of scenery and in a strange environment. Only when labour is well established and advanced is it more difficult to disturb its course and it is less likely that you fall prey to unnecessary intervention such as a syntocinon drip or pain relief.

Plan B – Emergency Birth Plan

Admittedly, my plan B was always simple. Due to a lack of homebirth midwives in Sweden, where I had three of my four freebirths, there was only one option for a true emergency: to go to the hospital, 30 minutes away. As the likelihood of encountering a true emergency however was extremely small in my case (I was healthy, had uncomplicated pregnancies and normal births) I didn't unduly worry about this. I somehow knew that things would go ok and I would not need plan B.

During my forest birth, I carried a mobile phone I used to call my husband once the baby was born.

In countries with more midwives available it is easier to find one to call upon in the case of doubts. Some midwives are happy supporting freebirthing women. If you wish to have a midwife as back up, discuss all the details with her before the baby's birth.

It is definitely preferable to have a trusted midwife to call upon to avoid a potentially unnecessary hospital transfer and having to deal with hospital staff not supportive of freebirth as well as the outside influence and patronising environment you were seeking to avoid in the first place.

In summary, I don't think you can ever have the perfect emergency plan. Depending on personal preference and need for a safety net, every woman has to make provisions for her individual situation.

This might be an exhaustive list of birth preferences and things you definitely want to avoid in case of transfer, the knowledge that the hospital bag is packed with everything needed, the car has a full tank of petrol and is ready on the drive and/or someone is available to drive you if necessary.

In this context it is probably helpful to find out why freebirths transfer to the hospital in reality. There are large collections of birth stories on internet sites such as www.unassistedchildbirth.com and www.birthjunkie.com.

Most planned freebirths happen at home as intended. The most common reason for transfer seems to be a placenta that doesn't want to come out or is slow to do so, yet does come out with some help in the hospital. Another fairly frequent reason is fear or panic in the mother or one of the members of her family.

Both of these reasons for transfer can be traced back to a lack of preparation. There are some reports of medically necessary transfers due to a morbidly adherent placenta or a uterine rupture after a previous caesarean section. Those are rare however.

The legal side

Births that intentionally happen without a midwife present are not covered under the law in any country that I know of. It follows that planned or accidental freebirth is not a punishable offence.

In Germany, doctors and other health professionals have a duty to consult a midwife when attending a birth. But this does not apply to women who may birth so quickly that they don't have time to get a midwife to attend. And whether a freebirth was intended or accidental is difficult to prove after the fact. When a supporter during an unattended birth becomes actively involved in helping with the birth in a professional capacity, is not clearly defined. In Germany, cases of this have so far never reached court.

In Austria the situation is slightly different. The midwives' law § 3 (BGBl. No. 310/1994, from the 25/2/2014) dictates that a pregnant woman has to consult a midwife for her birth. Which is very odd as a midwives' law should not prescribe what a normal pregnant citizen has to do. I don't know of any cases in which an Austrian woman has had to defend her decision not to consult a midwife for birth and postnatal care in court.

There is no law that disallows freebirth or makes it a duty to consult a midwife in Switzerland.

In the UK, a woman has the right to appropriate medical care during a homebirth. This means in general she will be provided with a midwife. Still in some cases the hospital may well deem an ambulance sent to the address as appropriate. There is no legal obligation to consult a midwife though. Theoretically the woman's partner can be prosecuted under the law if he is deemed to have 'played' midwife, even if he was in a different room during the birth. I can only think of one case where this has led to a monetary fine.

The Nursing and Midwifery Council have recently given out very clear guidance on the legal situation regarding freebirthing in the UK and state:

"Free birthing' is legal as long as the birth is not attended or the responsibility for care is not assumed or undertaken by an 'unqualified individual'. An 'unqualified individual' is a person who is not a registered doctor or midwife but acts in that capacity during birth. The woman assumes full responsibility for her child's birth, but she may and can have her partner, a relative or a friend present in a supportive role. If a woman chooses not to contact or engage a midwife it is her right to do so.'

Their very extensive guidance can be read here in its entirety:

www.nmc-uk.org/Nurses-and-midwives/Regulation-in-practice/Regulation-in-Practice-Topics/Free-birthing1

Similar conditions apply in Australia, New Zealand, the USA and most other countries.

The chapter for men, by men

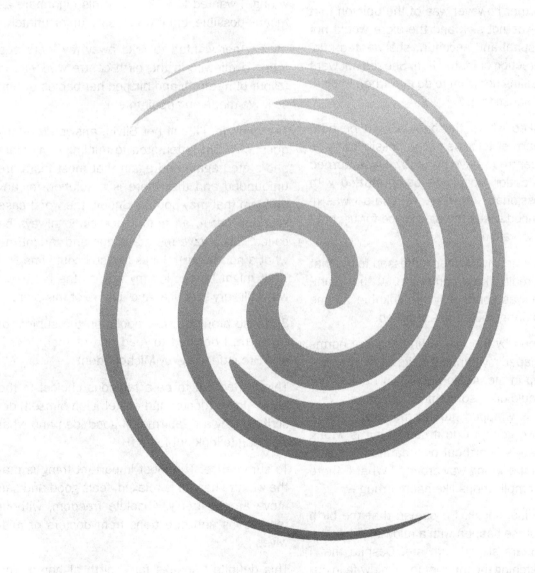

Our journey to freebirth, together

Marco talks about his experience.

Dedicated to my true love, whose stubborn streak let me experience the most beautiful moment of my life!

While anticipating the birth of our baby, the question of place of birth came up at some point. In the hospital of course, in my opinion. I have to admit, alternatives were absolutely no option for me. My partner however was of the opinion that firstly she was not sick and therefore would not need a hospital and secondly, she wanted support, not direction or instruction. She did not want strangers telling her what to do and when to do it. That made sense to me.

When I asked where the baby should be born then, my partner told me of the possibility to go to a birth centre to have our baby. I was worried about this option despite it being staffed with birth professionals. After several chats I was finally convinced it was the right place for us, but I still had reservations.

After some time, my partner confessed to me that she would really like a homebirth. At that point, this option was completely unthinkable for me and far too dangerous. I was shocked.

Fears, formed by the media and societal norms that had shaped my thinking in life up to now kept bubbling up in me. Again and again I asked her what we would do if 'something happened'. What if the cord is wrapped around the baby's neck? What are we going to do if something is wrong with the baby's heartbeat or breathing? What if the baby is the wrong way around? What if there are other complications like haemorrhage?

After the initial shock, I assumed that the birth would of course happen with a midwife in attendance. My fears stayed with me. Despite that I started searching the internet for a midwife in our area who would support homebirths.

But my partner craftily kept me from calling her repeatedly, until she finally told me: 'I DON'T WANT A MIDWIFE WITH ME WHEN I GIVE BIRTH, I WANT TO DO IT ALONE.'

Alone. That would mean that I would have to help her. And our six year old son would be there. NO – unimaginable! PANIC! The rug was pulled from under my feet. Me, who knows nothing about birth and who is even worried about complications occurring in the hospital! Never! No way! I would never be able to forgive myself if something went wrong. I wanted to wake from this nightmare as fast as possible, but it was reality, unfortunately.

My partner wanted to take away my fears and found a midwife in the birth centre who was in favour of freebirth and birthed her babies by herself. We made an appointment.

The midwife, I'll call her Silvia, answered all my questions. She attempted to minimise my fears and stated again and again that most fears are unfounded and that there is a solution for any problem that may pop up. Should the worst case scenario occur, an ambulance could always be called. Silvia gave me many tips and taught me what a normal birth looks like so I could imagine what might be coming my way on the big day. I was still very sceptical and unsure of this plan.

She also brought a few books on the subject of freebirth. I decided to read one of them, 'Birth and Breastfeeding' by Michel Odent.

This turned out to be a fabulous choice! In the book, Odent (doctor and obstetrician himself) describes, why a freebirth is a good idea and what we need to look out for.

To summarise: The most important thing is that the woman herself is relaxed, feels good and can move around freely. Absolute freedom, without restrictions and directions from doctors or midwives.

This definitely speaks for a birth at home. The partner's job is preparing the home and fulfilling his partner's every need predominantly. Relaxed woman, relaxed baby – according to Odent.

Perhaps some of you are afraid of passing out or not being able to manage in other ways. Birth is often very painful for women and I, too, struggled to see my partner in pain without being able to relieve it. But apart from that, everything went fantastically! There were no complications. And during those hours of birth I was so focussed on supporting my partner that I never thought of the 'what ifs'.

I would advise any sceptical men to go with a freebirth if their partner really wants to have one. I will remember the moment I guided my daughter into the world with my own two hands forever and always and I am incredibly proud of myself and my partner as she did such an amazing job.

On the subject of fear, I can only say: Once we had made the decision for a freebirth we have only ever thought that everything would go well. We didn't have any negative thoughts. Nature knows what it is doing and it did. At the end of the day we are only mammals and they generally manage without hospital, anaesthesia etc.

Also, trust your baby! It will come when it wants to. And don't worry, it knows the way.

'I could not manage to get rid of my fears.'

About the role of the support person during freebirth.

Linus talks about his experience.

I became afraid for the first time when I had trouble hearing the baby's heartbeat. Labour had been going on for two, maybe three hours and the little one hadn't moved for some time. I had always believed that you didn't need to listen to the heartbeat if the baby is moving.

But now I was starting to worry and got nervous. A little later he moved again and the fear disappeared. The birth progressed slowly, much slower than the first birth I had experienced. We were both very tired. He was eventually born (after about 6 hours, so the birth wasn't that long after all) and when I held him I was initially very happy. But then the fear resurfaced again, properly this time. Our daughter had complained loudly immediately after her birth.

But the baby I was now holding did not do anything and looked very blue indeed. In that moment, many thoughts went through my head, none of them positive. It took maybe 20 seconds until he started crying, but those moments I was holding this oddly blue looking and lifeless baby in my arms felt like a very very long time. Luckily everything was fine. Retrospectively it was a very tiring birth but ultimately positive and beautiful. My partner had no tears and although the baby was 16 days overdue by the doctor's calculations, he did not look overdue in the slightest.

During the third birth I was present at (and our second without a midwife), everything happened quickly again. Differently to the other births, my partner seemed doubtful that everything would turn out well. She said things like: 'I can't do it anymore.' and screamed 'I want a break, not yet!' This time it wasn't single moments that were particularly scary, but my fear and worry were with me all the time, and certainly in the last hour of the birth (which lasted about 2.5 hours altogether).

I had the feeling that something wasn't quite right, and the baby was maybe in the wrong position. We did indeed think afterwards that the baby came through the birth canal with its head tipped to one side. Additionally, it seemed to me like something was in front of the head when it became visible and palpable for the first time. The head moved back up again and then started to advance properly with the next contraction. Perhaps the cord or a hand had been in front of the head. Everything turned out to be fine with this birth as well. But I did need quite some time to recover from the fear and stress.

I generally don't think you should approach the subject of freebirth with fear in mind. Quite the opposite: It is important to imagine how normal the birth can be if it goes the way the pregnant woman wants it to. And it is especially important to remember that fear actually 'makes' birth difficult.

Why am I focussing on fear then? To answer that question I have to explain a little more about the role the support person, such as boyfriend, female friend, mother, father or others, takes at the birth.

One of the most common questions I was asked when people found out about our plans to freebirth was: 'Who caught the baby?' Apart from the basic misunderstanding that a second person is required for this, it also implies the question about the supporter taking the role of the midwife.

This continues when it comes to questions about the cord, but also other practical issues such as disposal of the placenta and so on. The assumption that one takes over the classic midwife duties during an unattended birth is not wrong on the whole of course.

However, because freebirthing means having made the conscious decision not to have a midwife present, it seems somewhat counterproductive in most cases for the supporter to play midwife.

So how does the role of the midwife differ from the role of the partner during freebirth, or even better, how should it differ? In most cases, it is different on two points. Firstly, the relationship with the birthing mother is closer and more intimate. Secondly, and this is likely the biggest difference for most freebirthers, it is often not clear anymore who has the power to make decisions when a midwife is present. Decisions have to be discussed and the birthing woman not only has to deal with her birth, but also with the midwife.

If you attend a birth as a layperson, you need to accept the pregnant woman as holding complete authority when it comes to all things concerning birth. To keep the birth as pleasant as possible, you should refrain from trying to influence any decision in which the mother is not involving you in the first place.

From my point of view – as friend and father, who has supported two freebirths – this acceptance is the most difficult part for the birth partner as I had the feeling again and again that a change in position during birth would make sense.

You might even think that a doctor should be called. The conflict arising from this is very acute and difficult in that particular situation. Do I disregard my girlfriend's wishes because I think I can see something she can't? The answer should generally be 'no'. And this is where fear comes into play.

I really don't believe there are many supporters who do not feel afraid at any point during the birth. Fear that something 'bad' may happen, injury to mother or baby, or worse. And the fear that you should have done something, like call the midwife or even an ambulance.

But in the vast majority of cases this fear is unfounded, and this is true of most fears. My girlfriend told me after our second freebirth that she never had doubts during the births that everything would be all right. I felt completely different. Had I started a discussion about if and who to call for help during my moments of doubt, I probably would have made the birth much more difficult for her.

Of course I don't mean a quick question for reassurance but letting go of it in case she says everything is fine. It is difficult to accept my girlfriend as the absolute expert as the situation is such an unusual one. A woman who cannot speak for the pain, possibly dehydrated, bent over in agony and possibly locking herself in the bathroom, may look to you like someone who cannot make rational decisions. It might seem sensible to make decisions for her, although you are not thinking clearly either due to fear.

The mixture of your own fear and the sense that the birthing woman might not be able to make sensible decisions may lead you to interfere and ruin the freebirth in a sense. In this situation, your own judgement, with some certainty, is worse than that of a midwife, for two reasons:

Firstly you are lacking the medical knowledge of a midwife and secondly you don't have the experience, which means a midwife is less likely to act out of fear.

Of course there are exceptions in which it is a good thing to call for help. In the case of haemorrhage the birthing woman may be so weakened from blood loss that she is truly unable to judge the situation appropriately. This is exceedingly rare though. In most cases though, your own fear is the biggest danger to a successful freebirth and if you try to interfere, you are likely to encounter a confrontation with the birthing woman. And this confrontation can make birth more dangerous and affect your long term relationship negatively. Remember that the desire for a freebirth is generally a desire for autonomy. And this autonomy needs to be unconditionally accepted by the birth partner.

So, after three births, two of those freebirths, my most important piece of advice for fathers to be is to discuss all potential scenarios BEFORE the birth and clearly define your role:

When do you want me to step in?

What are the limits?

What if I don't want to be part of a certain decision? Do I leave the birthing woman alone? Or is it especially important then to accept and live with the decision 100% ?

You should also consider if you feel able to be there in a solely supporting role, or if you perhaps don't want to be a birth partner. The pregnant person also needs to consider this. Does she feel her partner would be able to 'just watch'?

Many people are put off discussing these questions because of the potential conflict this discussion may cause, but it really is better to clear up these issues BEFORE the birth rather than DURING, when it might not only influence the birth negatively but also has potential for huge conflict in your relationship.

In this sense, I would like to invite you to talk through any scenarios mentioned earlier and anything you may feel unsure about during a birth. We did this, however not in the depth that I am advising you to do this now, to make a beautiful birth as likely as possible.

On the whole though, our births were the most beautiful events in my life so far, despite all the doubts and fears.

When the midwife makes a mistake – an interview

Despite homebirths having a great reputation when it comes to the mother's satisfaction, they don't always happen without issues. I have experienced this myself as have others.

This is an aspect that becomes clear in many women's plans for freebirth: a birth professional interfered in a previous birth, and she wants to keep this birth as unhindered as possible.

Urs tells his story.

How did you come to plan a birth without midwives?

Urs: Our first son was born at home with a midwife present. The birth went well, but there were problems with the placenta. The midwife pulled the placenta out after about 10–12 minutes which led to a substantial blood loss for my wife, which was not without danger.

We could not understand how an experienced homebirth midwife would intervene in such a way. We were so surprised. My wife felt betrayed. This is why she decided on a freebirth when the midwife threatened intervention during her second pregnancy. The midwife scared her and told her it would be dangerous if she started bleeding again.

I accepted my wife's decision without objections as we knew what had really caused my wife's bleeding. The midwife did not think that her premature intervention was to blame for the haemorrhage.

What fears, thoughts and expectations did you have with regards to the next birth?

Urs: I hoped that it would go well this time if we gave the placenta the time it needed to separate by itself. I didn't worry about the birth or the baby as I had confidence the outcome would be good.

How did you experience the birth yourself?

Urs: I felt at ease with just the two of us in a homely and intimate atmosphere. The birth happened in the early hours of the morning, when our older son was still asleep. I found it relaxing to witness the birth of our child unfolding naturally without outside influence and intervention.

What was your role during the birth?

Urs: I prepared everything so that my wife could birth our baby in optimal conditions. Amongst other things this included filling the birthpool with water at a comfortable temperature. I also made sure the room was warm and cozy and brought everything my wife was asking for.

I cooled her brow and gave her drinks. She didn't seek or need any physical contact, neither did she need any mental support.

I could not do much but create the best external conditions for birth.

What expectations came true?

Urs: If you leave birth, including afterbirth, alone, it works beautifully. Fears block the normal process of birth. Birth is one of the most natural things in the world and if you accept the process with trust and self confidence as we did, it can be a powerful and wonderful event, even without hospital and intervention and all the issues those can bring.

Many interventions such as caesareans happen because women have been made afraid and don't trust their own ability to birth their babies. They believe birth is not possible without intervention anymore.

What surprised you during the birth?

Urs: We had one homebirth with a midwife and two freebirths. With the latter two I was surprised how quickly the births happened.

How did your friends and family react to your plans for birth without a midwife?

Urs: We had comments like: 'You are brave, we would never feel able to do this.' Or: 'If something happens and you are not in hospital, what then? Our baby/mother would have died if the doctor hadn't been able to come so quickly.' Or: 'It is irresponsible to birth a baby at home, alone.' Or: 'We could see ourselves having a baby in the birth centre but not all alone, at home.'

What advice would you give other fathers to be?

Urs: I would say, leave the decision where to birth the baby to the woman. She is the one who has to be at ease during the birth. It makes sense to inform yourself about all the alternatives to hospital birth.

The baby is born

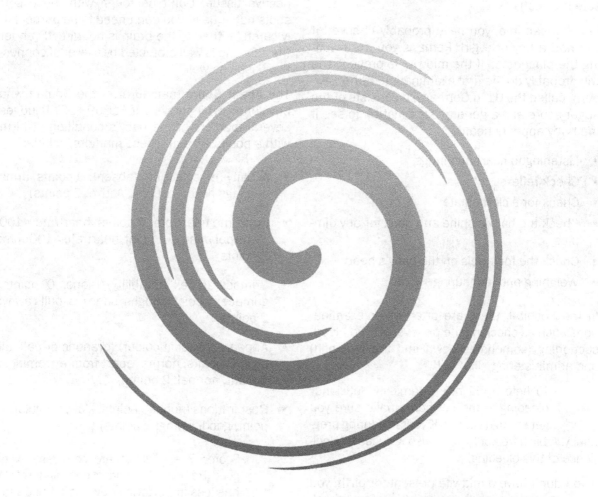

The first hour with your newborn

And then you suddenly hold it in your arms: your child! It is looking at you with big eyes and you look back. Love at first sight.

Your baby recognises your voice from its time in your belly, it knows your smell – apparently amniotic fluid smells of you – and soon it is suckling at your breast as if it had always done it. (Please be aware of good attachment and positioning from the start to avoid sore nipples!)

In the meantime, you have probably checked if you had a boy or a girl. Perhaps you are awaiting the placenta.....if the midwife is present she will probably do the first examination of the newborn, called the U1 in Germany. It consists of the Apgar score and a general examination to see if the baby appears healthy:

- Listening to heart and lungs
- Check reflexes
- Check for a cleft palate
- Check the baby's spine and back for any dimples
- Check the fontanels on the baby's head
- Weighing and measuring

In the hospital, there are often other examinations such as checking the pH level of cord blood, suctioning (sometimes down into the stomach) and administering Vitamin K.

To help avoid rare Vitamin K deficiency bleeding in the newborn, make sure you get enough vitamin K yourself during pregnancy. A birth free of trauma also reduces the incidence of this bleeding.

If you don't have a midwife present for birth, you can make sure your baby is well yourself and check if there are any obvious abnormalities. Weighing and measuring (length and head circumference) are easily done with things you already have at home. A measuring tape as is used to measure fabric is a good tool here.

If you don't have baby scales, just stand on the scales with and without your baby and calculate your baby's weight from the difference.

The big fontanel is a coin sized soft spot on the babies head, just above the hairline towards the front. It can visibly pulsate as long as it is still present (it ossifies gradually towards the end of the second year of life). If it seems to bulge inwards, it may signal dehydration in the baby.

The small fontanel is located on the back of the baby's head, a few fingers width above the nape of the neck. Both fontanels are covered with connective tissue. Don't be rough with these soft spots but equally, you don't need to be particularly careful either as the brain is not directly under the skin and is well protected by a layer of connective tissue as well.

The **Apgar Score** (named after the woman who developed it, Virginia Apgar *1909 +1974) judges several markers of the baby's condition at birth with a points system. These markers include:

- **A**ctivity (muscle tone) (absent: 0 points, arms and legs flexed: 1 point, Active: 2 points)

- **P**ulse (no heartrate: 0 points, heartrate <100 beats per minute: 1 point, heartrate >100bpm: 2 points)

- **G**rimace (reflex irritability) (none: 0 points, grimace: 1 point, coughs, sneezes, pulls away: 2 points)

- **A**ppearance (skin colour) (cyanotic or pale all over: 0 points, normal apart from extremities: 1 point, normal: 2 points)

- **R**espirations (none: 0 points, slow, irregular: 1 point, good, crying: 2 points)

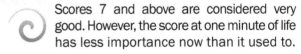

Scores 7 and above are considered very good. However, the score at one minute of life has less importance now than it used to.

Should you birth by yourself, you are unlikely to measure time and give out points anyway. You are hardly going to suction your baby, hospital style, just to get the baby to give a vigorous cry. But if you are in any doubt, the Apgar score can be a good guide for a rough evaluation of your baby's condition.

By the way, a baby who does not cry is not necessarily unwell. Quite the opposite: many babies who are born without trauma don't feel the need to cry right after birth. If you feel your baby's heart beating, it looks quite rosy and is breathing with some regularity, all is generally well.

It is normal for the baby ...

- ... to look bluey-pink in the first few minutes.
- ... not to breathe for the first minute when the cord is still pulsing.
- ... to make some noises while breathing in the first 20 minutes
- ... to have bluey hands and feet and even head in the first 1–2 hours of life.

But keep your baby warm and covered according to temperature, as blue skin discolouration from cold is absolutely not necessary.

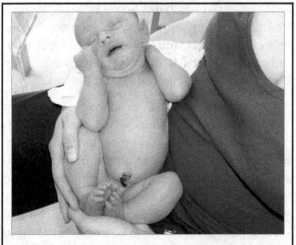

3 days old: our second son, cord stump still attached. As you can see, he still likes to be in the position he was in for the nine months in my belly.

Breastfeeding and the family bed

You can assume that every woman can breast-feed as long as she has healthy breasts and is well in herself and not malnourished.

In the first few days there won't be much milk, despite the baby's vigorous suckling. Don't limit this stimulation, for several reasons:

For one, the baby can learn to drink at the breast before your milk comes in, which makes your breasts very full and the nipples harder to grasp.

And secondly, it gets to suckle colostrum (yellow to orange in colour), the special first milk, full of protein and antibodies.

Between the third and fifth day, you will undergo a transformation that might make a page 3 girl envious. You will never again have breasts as big as this (unless you have another baby), so: if you want, take pictures of that magical moment when your milk comes in for the first time!

Breastfeeding often enters a critical phase at this point. Your breasts are full to bursting and tight as a drum and your baby may find it hard to latch and take in all of the nipple and areola. Furthermore, your nipples are not used to the constant demands of a suckling baby.

So bear with it for a while. Having plenty of skin to skin contact with the baby certainly makes the start of breastfeeding easier. And if you persevere, things soon become easier and you will (hopefully) forget all about the difficult early days.

Sore nipples can benefit from lanolin ointment, which can be applied before and after feeds without needing to be washed off. A very engorged breast can be relieved with gentle massage towards the nipple in a hot shower, which should make latching the baby easier.

In case you are dealing with a temporary oversupply, be careful with expressing milk as this suggests increased demand for milk to your body and it will ramp up production and make even more – too much – milk.

In the next weeks and months you will go through phases again and again when it seems like your baby wants to feed frequently or even almost permanently. This is not a sign you are not making enough milk. Those phases are growth spurts where the baby's requirements for breastmilk increase. By suckling frequently, the baby signals your body to start making more milk to match those requirements.

If you have doubts about the ability of your breasts, don't supplement too early, as this can produce the exact problem you are worried about. Think about it: Your breasts only ever make as much milk as your baby demands.

If its belly gets filled by other means like a bottle of formula, it won't 'order' enough milk by suckling at your breast and you might end up supplementing long term.

Should your milk production seem low despite plenty of skin to skin, breastfeeding on demand and good nutrition, the problem may be hypothyroidism, other hormonal problems (such as polycystic ovary syndrome or an unknown insulin resistance) or even some remnants of placenta still present in the uterus. The latter generally makes itself known by recurring, heavy vaginal bleeding though.

Your doctor can rule out the above causes for low milk supply. Gentle remedies that support milk production are traditionally so called 'mother's milk' teas, malt beer and barley 'coffee'. Fenugreek and Blessed Thistle (in the form of capsules perhaps) as well as homeopathy (for example Phytolacca) can be used for the same purpose.

When there is legitimate fear that the baby may not be getting enough nutrition, a top up meal with another mother's milk, goat's milk or even formula may be helpful.

Are you getting good breastfeeding advice? If you know a breastfeeding counsellor, an experienced midwife or have a good friend with positive breastfeeding experience, their knowledge can be invaluable.

However, there are many pieces of advice that can make your breastfeeding journey unnecessarily complicated: Only ever one breast per feeding? Always empty the breast completely, even if you need to pump to do so? Only ever feed once every 3–4 hours? Stop breastfeeding after a certain time? Only breastfeed at certain times, and not during the night? Wean off the breast at 6 months, a year at the latest? And never nurse your baby to sleep?

Of course there will eventually be some sort of rhythm and your baby will want feeding every few hours. But most babies get hungry during the night just as much as during the day, and as soon as they hit a growth spurt (and there are rather a lot of those in the first few weeks) this rhythm goes to pot again completely. And of course you can give your baby only one breast per feed but surely if the baby is still hungry after that, you will also offer the second one.

How long a baby takes at the breast until satisfied varies from baby to baby. Some efficient feeders are done within minutes while some connoisseurs take longer. You will soon figure out what makes your child tick, when it is hungry and when it is crying for an entirely different reason.

Sometimes your child might only want to suckle for comfort and can't deal with your milk ejection reflex. In those circumstances your little finger or a dummy might make appropriate substitutes. Gently expressing by hand (which, by the way, you can practice in pregnancy when you might already produce some milk) and feeding from a cup or glass can also help to give traumatised (sore) nipples a bit of a break to enable healing.

It is very convenient to be able to nurse your baby in the night without having to transfer it to a different sleep environment. This is easiest if your baby sleeps right next to you, with no barriers.

To give everyone plenty of room to rest comfortably, an extra wide mattress (we like 1.20m for mum and baby), placed on the floor so the baby can't fall far, works very well. You should place some bed slats underneath so that moisture does not cause damage to the floor or the mattress. For all beds of normal height, solutions to stop a baby from falling off, such as a bed guard, are available widely.

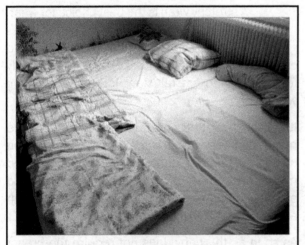

Our family bed solution, three metres wide. There is now – just about – room for 4 children and mother.

So how long can you keep your baby with you during the night? Doesn't it have to learn to fall asleep alone and without suckling at the breast?

If you would like to avoid frustration and keep a trusting bond between you and your baby, wait until your child is ready. Don't be disappointed though if that turns out to be much later than society has you believe.

Research by anthropologist Katherine A. Dettwyler concludes that the natural weaning age for humans is somewhere between 3 and 7 years of age. In societies in which children are able to nurse as long as they want, weaning starts to happen around 3 to 4 years old, no stress or frustration. Of course those children are not ex-

clusively breastfed for all that time but they still drink from their mother's breast when they can walk. They also generally still prefer to sleep in their mother's bed to sleeping alone at 1, 2, 3 or more years of age.

My tip for you: Please free yourself from your expectations about what your baby should be able to do at which point in time as soon as possible. Accept your particular set of circumstances and choose the way that seems best for your family, especially you and your baby.

Even when you are pregnant again, your breastfeeding relationship doesn't have to come to a close, if you don't want it to. I have breastfed the older siblings in all subsequent pregnancies. This does not pose a risk to a healthy pregnancy, though nipples can at times be rather sensitive. It is extremely convenient to have an older child around when your milk comes in to relieve engorgement efficiently. And it can also help to avoid jealousy towards the new brother or sister.

Please keep an extra close eye on your own nutrition, so you don't give more than you have or are taking in. Feeding two children at the same time is called tandem feeding and mostly known from women feeding twins.

In this context I will mention the safety of a family bed with regards to 'Sudden infant death syndrome (SIDS)':

Bed sharing is a subject much argued about by experts and is sometimes portrayed as a risk factor for SIDS, even if the parents don't smoke, take drugs or drink alcohol. On the other hand bedsharing is a common practice worldwide and well recognised and normal in countries such as Japan.

Around 60% of Japanese people state that they share a bed with their babies while only about 16% of Americans say so. In reality though, bed sharing seems to be far more common than it seems at first glance. More specific data collection showed that 26% of all babies either shared their parents bed either 'always' or 'nearly always'. (Whiting 1981)

It appears that the social taboo around bed sharing leads parents to fudge their answers. And even though many more children bedshare with their parents in Japan, their SIDS rate is around 0.2 – 0.3 in 1.000 births. In the US, the rate is 0.5 in 1.000. (McKenna 2007)

The optimal family bed should be sufficiently big and have a firm mattress. The baby should be protected from falling out of the bed or into the gap in the middle (also called the visitor's gap in Germany), and strangulation hazards should be eliminated.

Sudden Infant Death Syndrome is defined as the sudden and unexplained death of a child in the first but also up to the end of the second year of life. Most cases occur in the first 6 months of life. The most common period for sudden infant death is between the second and fourth month of life.

A certain amount of protection against SIDS is provided by breastfeeding, the baby sleeping on its back, but also by sleeping with its mother in a room that is free of smoke and not too warm. Babies do sometimes have small pauses in their breathing and that is not abnormal. The mother's breathing rhythm stimulates the baby to breathe more regularly and with less pauses. (McKenna 2005)

There is some evidence that there are more frequent irregularities in a baby's breathing rhythm in the days after the diphtheria/whooping cough/tetanus vaccination, which is routinely given to small babies. (Scheibner 1991)

Carrying, swaddling and calming

You can usually avoid buying an unwieldy pram by investing in a couple of good slings or wraps. Initially, your baby is likely to want to be close to you anyway and when the baby is around 6 months old and can sit by itself, it can either be carried still or you can start using a good folding pushchair. The latter are also easily fitted in the boot of a average sized car.

A stretchy wrap is the best choice for wearing a newborn. Later, when the baby has got better muscle tone, a soft structured carrier is also suitable and easy to use, especially for fathers who are reluctant to handle a 5 long wrap sling.

It is likely best to try out the slings at one of the many locally available sling libraries before you decide on a particular model. Personally I carried my children in a wrap (classic woven wrap and african Kanga) and in a homemade Mei Tai from around 6 months of age.

As soon as the baby does not require the breast as frequently, it is worth starting to backcarry. It is gentle on the mother's spine and it is easier to get on with household chores when the baby is safely tucked on mother's back rather than in front. In traditional cultures, babies are more often than not carried on backs.

Babywearing is also a wonderful tool for babies reluctant to sleep. With the right sling and some practice you can put the child down on a bed for extended naps or, if the baby fell asleep in the car, carry on with the sling without waking it up.

Another method for calming babies is swaddling. In many pictures you can see Jesus in his cradle, swaddled. Swaddling means wrapping a baby securely in a suitable piece of fabric with its arms close to its body so movement is restricted. In modern times this practice has slowly got a bad reputation as babies used to be swaddled for

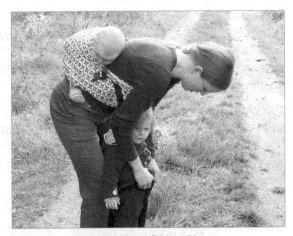

Babywearing with the African Kanga.

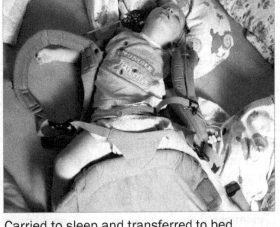

Carried to sleep and transferred to bed.

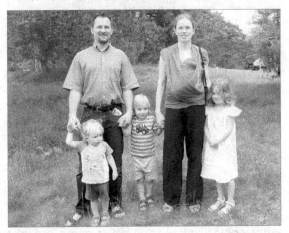

Our family with newborn in a 5.2m wrap.

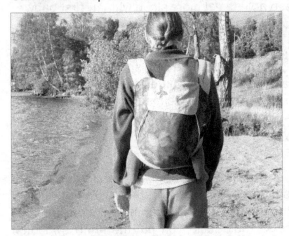

Baby in homesewn Mei Tai.

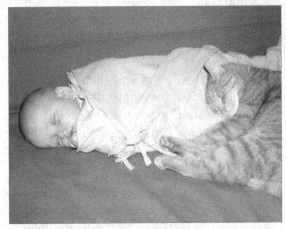

A swaddled baby sleeps well. The hand (pushed out of the swaddle while asleep) should not be visible.

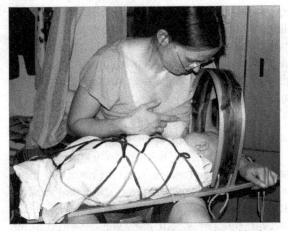

Mobile bed swaddle function: the Native American cradle board

long stretches and were not allowed to move, to the detriment of their development.

There has been a renewed interest in swaddling babies in recent years, and in the right doses it can be a great help. Especially small babies find it had to coordinate their arms and legs efficiently, yet they have many reflexes. One of those reflexes causes the sudden lifting of the arms in an exaggerated startle gesture (Moro reflex). Our first baby woke itself up hourly with this movement. As soon as our little mouse had gone to sleep, she would startle and the cycle of crying and trying to calm her would start anew.

If I had known then what I know now, I would have been able to get more sleep with my first baby.

While swaddled, babies feel safe and held, just like in their mothers bellies. Getting used to all the space in the extrauterine world takes some time and it is easily observed how quickly a baby calms once swaddled firmly. Babies tend to sleep well when swaddled. A part of my baby routine has always been: swaddle, feed, sleep.

During relentless growth spurts and when you are just too tired to carry a teething/ill/otherwise unsettled baby around, it can help to do what I call 'the swaddle rock': you put the firmly swaddled baby on its back and start rocking it from side to side. In small and fast or long and sweeping movements, whatever works best. Perhaps sing a lullaby while doing this. Even an exhausted mother can manage that in the middle of the night, even if she is too tired for anything else. The best thing about it: The success rate is high and you can stay in bed.

You can buy special swaddling cloths/blankets, but really, any large piece of thin material will do. In winter you can use a thin blanket even. You can also buy more structured swaddling garments that can be fastened with velcro. They do have to be the right size however, otherwise your baby will have too much room in them and not feel sufficiently secure. The need to keep buying more sizes as the baby grows makes this option fairly cost intensive.

Growth spurts

As already mentioned, every baby goes through phases of accelerated development. In the early days, several of these phases follow on each others heels.

The older the child, the less frequent these episodes – however, they don't become less intense. During these times, the baby's brain gets reprogrammed and 'recalibrated': suddenly it experiences its surroundings differently and can manage to turn over, propel itself forward and more.

These new and unusual impressions are difficult for the baby to process and this often results in crying and being unsettled.

So you can't always counteract a grumpy baby by giving the breast, toilet or change nappies. Sometimes you can only be there for your child, and calm, carry, swaddle and work together when the going gets tough. The reward comes afterwards: your child is calm again and suddenly has a new set of skills.

Pee and poo

What goes in at the top must come out at the bottom. The baby's first poop is green-brownish-black and very sticky indeed. It consists, amongst other components, of thick bile, swallowed hair, dead skin cells and the technical term for it is meconium.

To be able to get rid of this thick mass it is especially important the baby gets colostrum. The earlier the start of breastfeeding the quicker the baby will excrete this sticky stuff and the less chance there is for the development of a pathological form of newborn jaundice.

A certain level of jaundice is actually quite normal a few days after birth as the baby's body is breaking down fetal haemoglobin. The fetal haemoglobin is the red colouring of red blood cells, that has the ability to bind oxygen especially well. This enables the baby in utero to utilise oxygen from the mother optimally. After birth, this specific haemoglobin is not needed anymore and is broken down gradually.

During the breakdown of haemoglobin, the body firstly removes the central, oxygen binding heme which changes its original red colour, firstly into green (bile) and then to yellow bilirubin during further break down. This is responsible for the yellow skin and poo colour of a jaundiced newborn.

To stop the bilirubin being stored in the body and causing a pathological form of newborn jaundice, it has to go via the bile duct and into the gut to be excreted in faeces. So as long as breastfeeding gets established and works its laxative effects, the excretion of waste that leads to jaundice is ensured.

It will take about 2 or more years until your child will be able to go to the toilet himself. Until then you have several options for wee and poo containment that keep your carpets clean.

There is the modern classic, the **disposable nappy**. Put it on the baby, who fills it with poo or wee, then you dispose of it. Depending on age you will likely need between 4 to 7 nappies a day, for 2 or more years. This means having to buy nappies constantly and sending them to landfill for disposal.

Alternatively you can use **reusable nappies made from cloth**. They really don't take too much effort as cunning designs (elastic, velcro, inserts) make them very similar to the classic disposable nappy.

Money wise, cloth nappies are only good value when more than one child gets to use them, and you have to take into account the daily washing. But you don't have to buy nappies constantly and you don't put nappies in the bin.

And then there is what is known as **elimination communication** or **natural infant hygiene**.

Babies without nappies? How does that work?

Indeed it has worked worldwide for a long time before disposable and cloth nappies became available. Babies know from birth when they need to go, and send signals to let mothers know. Only when their natural instinct to signal elimination has been eradicated by super absorbent nappies do they start weeing and pooing without prior warning.

Is this how the myth of the immature sphincter came to be?

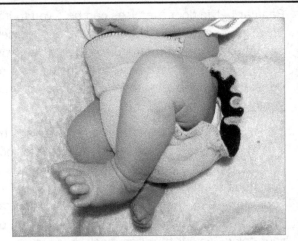

Home sewn fleece wrap with cotton inserts and flap for easy access for toileting.

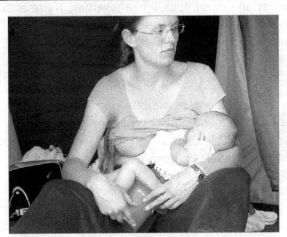

Even the smallest babies can be toileted on a tiny (Asia) potty (or a bush or a drain when out and about)

Countless observations in countries, where disposable nappies are uncommon or prohibitively expensive, show that babies, even newborns, know exactly when they need to go. If you tune in to their signals and give them frequent opportunities to eliminate, they will soon learn to hold on for longer or until an appropriate location for toileting is found.

So it is possible to catch wee and poo and therefore save using maybe not all, but certainly lots of nappies. The method is, however, not free of accidents and the success rate is very variable, depending on age of the baby and developmental leaps. So, letting the baby crawl on the expensive rug entirely without a nappy may not be recommended if you want to keep said rug clean, but certainly number twos can be caught reliably and hardly ever happen in a nappy if frequent opportunity for toileting is offered.

Cloth nappies are great as back up as the baby does not lose the connection between needing to go and wetness as they often do when wearing super absorbent disposable nappies. And because there will likely only be few incidences of a pooey nappy, the effort it takes to clean the wee soaked nappies is minimal.

Of course there are also mothers who remove all carpet and avoid back ups altogether. There are no limits to imagination and experimentation with this method.

For more detailed information on the subject of elimination communication there are plenty of websites and web forums as well as the following books: Infant Potty Training (Boucke 2008), Diaper Free: The Gentle Wisdom of Natural Infant Hygiene (Bauer 2006).

Your body before and after

The changes your body goes through after birth are just as spectacular as the changes during pregnancy.

In the first few days after birth your belly will look similar to a big soft pear. You will be able to see the 'pear' shrinking from day to day, and if you didn't put on too many pounds in pregnancy and were relatively fit before, you will soon look fairly non pregnant again.

You will however gain something else with regards to size: your boobs. A modest cup size A may grow to a D. Your old clothes may well fit around your belly again soon, but your increased cup size thwarts those plans, at least when it comes to nice close fitting tops.

You will notice another change, between your legs. Your pelvic floor can feel like a saggy hammock in the first few days after birth and certainly needs a few weeks to return to its original condition.

But fear not, only the first few days feel like your insides may actually fall out, and you might well not manage to walk for any length of time or carry anything heavier than your baby. And no one should be asking that of you anyway!

Regular pelvic floor exercises can help you to improve your pelvic floor. Nowadays Kegel exercises are generally recommended for this, where you tense your pelvic floor as if to stop the flow of urine and hold the tension for a few seconds until gently relaxing again.

However, solely doing Kegel exercises by themselves can actually make pelvic floor problems worse. A well functioning pelvic floor does not only rely on the muscles of the pelvic floor but also on the gluteal muscles and the ligaments that attach the pelvic floor to the bottom of your spine, similar to a hammock. If you do a lot of Kegel exercises and pull the 'back post of the hammock' (the bottom of your spine) forward with the tension in your pelvic floor, you may well have a strong pelvic floor. However, it will still sag as you moved one of its posts.

Pelvic floor dysfunction often arises from this combination: weak gluteal muscles plus lots of Kegeling.

For optimal results you should do plenty of deep squatting. For this, put your feet parallel, slightly over a shoulder width apart, keep your heels on the floor, your back relaxed, your eyes ahead and squat. Just the way countless people do in developing countries everyday as they don't have comfy chairs, sofas or toilets. In this deep squat, you are stretching the ligamentous attachment of your pelvic floor to the spine, while strengthening your pelvic floor and gluteal muscles, opening your whole pelvis.

For pelvic floor experts this new knowledge is revolutionary yet entirely logical. It comes from the American Katy Bowman, who is active on the internet as well as the author of a book. (Bowman 2013)

Rediscovering the classic squat not only helps you get back in shape after birth, it is also a great preparation for birth. Katy Bowman may exaggerate when she says: '300 squats a day will lead to an easy birth.' but she makes a point about the importance of a pelvis well trained with this method. It is likely that a pelvis accustomed to frequent squatting is one of the reasons why women of healthy traditional cultures often birth easily.

Another lovely way to be nice to your pelvic floor is trampolining and dancing. If you notice some urinary incontinence while doing either, take it as a sign that your pelvic floor could do with strengthening. Avoid exercises that put a great strain on your pelvic floor, especially if it is weak already. Gently bouncing on the trampoline without your feet taking off is enough to strengthen your core and pelvic floor.

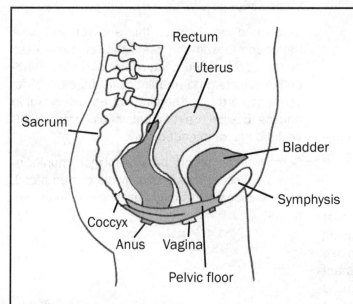

Figure 16: Female Pelvic floor
The pelvic floor is the elastic sling in the pelvic outlet, comprised of connective tissue and several different muscles.

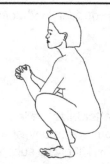

Figure 17: Squatting
Most adults have lost the ability to squat properly. Don't worry if you can't get all the way down initially. Go as low as comfortable – even if your bottom initially hovers half a meter over the floor. Practicing regularly will strengthen your pelvic floor and soon you will be able to do what comes easy to small children and people from developing countries: comfortably sit in a deep squat.

When you are feeling afterpains you can be sure that your uterus is working hard to return to its pre-pregnant state. You can feel this process happening via your abdominal wall. When your uterus disappears behind your symphysis pubis and into the pelvis, your uterus, the 'super organ' has pretty much gone back to its original size.

However, your abdominals may well be slightly separated still after several weeks and will benefit from gentle exercise to get back in shape.

Many small things that you have done countless times in your life have 'firsts' again after birth: the first wee, the first poo, the first time having sex again. Your lower belly and pelvis will still feel delicate and just 'different' for a while. Give yourself time, also in regards to the extra pounds you may be carrying. They will come in handy and help you provide ample amounts of milk in the next few months.

Once you feel mostly recovered, there is no reason for not doing regular exercise. Endurance, good posture – and everything that keeps your body fit – will contribute to your health in the long term, as long as you feel good doing it.

Lochia

The blood loss after birth (called lochia) will generally reduce from day to day, starting at the day of birth, when it will likely be substantially heavier than a period.

Lochia is accompanied by noticeable and sometimes unpleasant afterpains that are especially apparent when nursing your baby. These contractions of the uterus make sure that it shrinks back down to its pre-pregnant size and their intensity can sometimes be reduced by consciously releasing lochia into the toilet as the lochial blood can be trapped behind the now closed cervix and cause unpleasant pressure.

Lochia can continue for a while as spotting but it can also disappear for a while and recur after a few days with heavier flow. You might also find little clots or membranes that were left behind in the uterus after birth.

At 6 to 8 weeks after birth, the place where the placenta was implanted on the uterine wall should be healed, the uterus back to its original size and the lochia dried up. Until then you should rest as much as possible, the 'official postnatal period', the puerperium does last approximately this long for good reason.

Contrary to popular belief, lochia is not infectious unless you actually have an infection. Lochia does however contain bacteria, but not ones that make you ill. So, by all means, have a bath without fear of 'infecting' your nipples and baby or getting mastitis.

Sometimes bits of placenta remain in the uterus. This can happen occasionally even when the placenta appears complete and has not been pulled out of the uterus.

A warning sign for this scenario is long lasting or heavier lochia than normal in combination with uterine cramps and/or fever.

Ultrasound can confirm this and you will have the option to wait and see if the remnants pass by themselves. The doctor may prescribe methergine tablets (and antibiotics in the case of fever). Should the methergine not be successful in helping to expel the remnants of placenta, a D&C would be recommended.

Some women report passing bigger chunks of liver like tissue. This is usually old clotted blood, but occasionally this might also be placental remnants.

Hormones and emotions

Birth has released hormonal fireworks in your body, the side effects of which you are likely to feel for the following two days. You are on cloud nine and proud as punch of your amazing baby and your own achievement.

Then suddenly something changes within your body. You can usually tell initially from the sudden prolific supply of milk from your breasts that signals the abrupt hormonal changes in your body, also bringing the so called baby blues with them. If your birth was positive and happened in accordance with your wishes, you may only feel like crying for a day.

Let it out: milk, tears and lochia. You really could do without congestion in any of those three areas. Interestingly, they are all interconnected to a certain degree. Emotional stress can cause blocked milk ducts or, though much more rare, retained lochia.

The first few weeks with a newborn bring huge changes, especially if this is your first baby. Your daily and nightly rhythms are dictated by your baby's needs. You sit in your breastfeeding bubble, probably sleep deprived, and ask yourself if life will ever be different again, or in fact normal. Will you ever be able to shower again without one ear open for baby noises and not have to jump out of the shower dripping wet if you hear crying? When will you ever be able to sleep for a whole night again? And when will you be able to think straight again, without milk brain and sleep deprivation?

With regards to time, it is easy to lose your perspective, particularly with your first baby. It is hard to imagine that the initial 'caring for your baby round the clock phase' will only last a few months, that your baby will grow up incredibly fast and that every developmental leap is followed by a quieter phase.

So, don't be afraid! It will pass – and looking back, those times passed in a blink of the eye. Once your baby is not so tiny anymore, you can leave them with daddy or grandma for an hour of more. Then go out and do something for YOU! Let the fresh air blow the cob-webs away. You will love your family all the more for it.

Over the first few weeks your hormones and moods will balance out and you will start to be able to enjoy your new life more calmly. If this does not happen and you find it hard to feel positive towards your baby, please confide in someone trusted and if necessary, seek professional help.

"Well-meaning" advice from others

In the first few weeks you are definitely allowed to be selfish and decline visitors. If you need to, switch off your phone and ensure your calm postnatal period that way. The only thing that counts is whatever is good for you and your baby, pushy relatives will need to be patient. Personally, I did welcome visitors in the first few weeks but only if they brought food or cooked something for us.

You will not be able to avoid unsolicited advice. If it does not become overwhelming, just nod and smile. Advice is usually given with the best intentions, people naturally want to help.

However, if you feel yourself getting overwhelmed with all the 'helpful' advice, please vocalise this, firmly and politely. You will likely experience that people (often the older generation) become defensive and feel attacked personally when they see you do things very differently to them.

Being kind in a conciliatory manner can be of help here, but if you become too stressed, limit or don't allow visits by less than helpful advisors. You can use your partner as buffer if you find this conflict too exhausting. Give him clear instructions.

The comments of strangers might also be taken to heart and upset and unsettle you – especially if you are having your first baby and are feeling somewhat insecure still.

I always found it helpful to vent with my 'tribe' on suitable internet forums. What used to be the female community round the village well or in the sewing room can nowadays be found on the internet, and I have got to know many of the women in my internet tribe in real life. There might be no one like-minded around in real life, but they are only a click away in cyberspace.

Official business: Registering the birth

Most country's laws theoretically allow parents to register their baby's birth without input from a professional. However, many reports confirm that in reality, you will be viewed with scepticism and most authorities will demand a letter from an expert. But really, this is unnecessary.

Laws generally state that anyone who has knowledge that the birth has taken place can give notification of it. So, before you start your hunt for a birth certificate and get passed from pillar to post in the registry office, it is worth making some preparations:

- Call ahead of your actual visit to the registry office and explain the circumstances of your baby's birth. You can declare witnesses with regards to pregnancy and perhaps your partner can be direct witness of the birth. If there is no specific form for freebirths (as expected), it should be sufficient for you as the mother to draft a letter confirming the date, time and location of the birth. Your partner can witness and sign this document.

- If 'official proof' is requested anyway, it is easiest to ask a sympathetic midwife to sign a document to confirm your baby's date, time and location of birth. This midwife does not have to have provided your antenatal care, she simply needs to be prepared to sign off the birth notification. So you can ask any midwife at all, unless you have one as back up anyway.

- Of course you can also ask the registrar to show you the law that states those requirements in writing. Usually this will be impossible.

Self-directed Mothering

You have now learned about self-directed decision making. But you are still right at the start of your tiny baby's life and many decisions still have to be made by you. And it is still rather exciting to see how many of our societal myths need to be uncovered and overcome.

In the search for the path that is right for your family, always think about this rule of thumb: 'Does it feel right?' Don't ever let yourself be pushed into something that you can't truly agree with or that makes you feel doubtful in any way.

Inform yourself, and decide on the option that you agree with wholeheartedly, be it with regards to nighttime parenting, breastfeeding duration, vaccinations, dealing with illness, deciding on childcare or schooling.

There is a lot to come. But you are a strong woman and – hopefully with the support of family and friends – you will be able to deal with whatever life throws at you.

When will you have the next one?

Did you find lots of joy in your pregnancy and birth? Are you enjoying your amazing baby? Do you want the same health and optimal development for your next baby? If so, it might be worthwhile to wait a bit until you get pregnant again.

Weston Price, the dentist and researcher you read about earlier in this book, looked at siblings with regards to physical development and health. He found that in families following a Western diet, the closer a sibling was born to the bottom of the sibling order, the more deviation from optimal physical development as well as the more incidence of illness and malformation.

In Western countries, we often blame certain diseases on the age of the mother. However, it seems plausible that age is not the factor to blame but perhaps the increasing lack of nutrients in the mother's body as the number of (closely spaced) pregnancies increases. This is why it is extremely important to be extra mindful of nutrition and have a break between pregnancies, especially if you are planning to have many children. Most parents who want many children also want them to be strong and healthy.

In this context, it is interesting to examine what sort of age gap was common in traditional cultures. Not only did these cultures not encounter many of the diseases common in Western countries now, but they also specifically prepared their girls and women for pregnancy with special diets and made sure of a certain age gap between pregnancies. All this to ensure healthy and strong offspring.

The gaps between pregnancies were generally ensured by long breastfeeding periods, abstinence and polygamy, and were usually between 18 months and 4 years long. The average was 3 years. (Morell 2013)

A pregnancy too close to the previous one is proven to have a detrimental effect on health and chance of survival of the new baby. Chances of a healthy sibling are highest when the gap between pregnancies is no shorter than 18 months and no longer than 5 years (Conde-Aqudelo 2006), so that the older child is at least 27 months or no older than around 6 years old at birth.

Of course I am not saying that all children are prone to illness if born outside these parameters. But it is wise to consider these facts during your family planning and take care of yourself as a mother and space pregnancies sensibly – for your own health and that of your future children.

Listening to yourself, it is pretty easy to determine when a break might be indicated. And then it is worth obeying your body and giving it some respite, despite the call of the hormones just before ovulation.

Luckily, these days we have better options for spacing pregnancies than polygamy or years of abstinence. If you want cheap and hormone free contraception, the natural family planning method may be for you and it can be used during lactation too. Observing your temperature upon waking in combination with the consistency of your cervical mucus can lead to a contraceptive success rate close to that of the pill if used correctly.

You can attend courses to learn this method or read very helpful books on that subject, for example 'Taking charge of your fertility' (Weschler 2006).

We have used this method for many years, very successfully, either to avoid or achieve pregnancy – whatever was appropriate at the time.

Freebirth – Mothers tell their stories

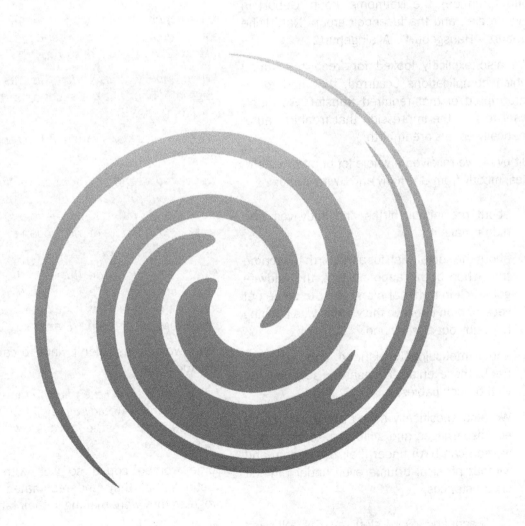

Call to action

The main part of this book was done by the beginning of 2014. My publisher and I decided spontaneously to also include the experiences of other mothers who have had a freebirth, as births without midwives are not that rare, really.

So we had a shout out on the internet to get women to contribute to this book. Of course we did this where freebirthers tend to congregate. Mainly on the homebirth forum (www.hausgeburtsforum.de), the Netmoms group 'Geburt in Eigenregie', and the facebook group 'Natürliche Geburt – Hausgeburt – Alleingeburt'.

We also explicitly looked for freebirths during which complications occurred, that had to be interrupted or that required transfer. We didn't want to give the impression that freebirth automatically equals dreambirth.

Bit by bit we received a whole lot of different stories, mostly from Germany and Switzerland:

- about precipitous births and midwives who didn't make it,

- about the secret wish for a freebirth that came true when birth happened fast, the midwife got stuck in traffic or didn't want to come out yet – or didn't believe the woman was pushing her baby out already and

- about meticulously planned and prepared freebirths, even after caesarean sections and with breech babies.

- We also specifically asked about self-directed miscarriages and stillbirths, to show how women can birth under their own steam and without physical trauma even under difficult circumstances.

Each and every story on the following pages is as unique as the people involved in it and their individual circumstances. It is very obvious how women's expectations have shaped their experiences.

The unplanned freebirth: When the baby is faster

For women who had their babies during an unplanned freebirth, the birth was often connected with a certain fear, insecurity and a longing for the midwife to turn up. Though all those births went well and without issues, women were very relieved and happy when their midwives did eventually turn up and took care of them.

The unplanned freebirths in this book all happened very quickly and unpredictably.

'Contractions came every 3–4 minutes at that point, but were only very gentle so I didn't think birth was imminent.' (Kathrin, 28)

'When I finally realised that this was not the first stage of labour but the second, everything went quickly'. (Uta, 35)

'My baby was born within 28 minutes from the first contraction.' (Beate, 41)

'We waited a long time for contractions after my waters went (about 12 hours) ... then suddenly some slightly painful contractions, nothing relevant for birth I thought, no reason to call the midwife ...' (Yvonne, 44)

'Finally I sat down on the bed, the naked little bundle in my arms. This is when U. (the midwife) entered the room. Now I could relax and she took care of everything else.' (Franziska, 37)

Some women just didn't want to call their midwife too early.

'I didn't want to call the midwife too early so that my contractions would stop again, so I just stayed in my bed and breathed joyously with every contraction.' (Franziska, 37)

Some women coped so well with their contractions that they underestimated how much progress they were making in their labour.

'The contractions were getting a little more intense, but were easy to cope with. Around 12.10 they were becoming painful and we called the midwives. A few contractions later I had the need to go to the toilet again. However, the need to

kneel in front of the sofa appeared to be stronger. With the next contraction I noticed that I didn't need the toilet after all ... my husband could already see the head.' (Kathrin, 28)

The transition from unplanned to a half planned freebirth is often smooth.

The half planned freebirth: When being alone turns out to be right

There is a middle ground between a completely unplanned freebirth and a meticulously planned out one: The woman dreams of a birth alone, but because it is usual to have a midwife present or because her partner is against a freebirth she calls on one anyway. Secretly though, she remains flexible on when to call the midwife or plays with the possibility that she may call her too late.

'The first thought about possibly birthing without a midwife present or maybe taking the 'risk' of calling her too late came early, at around 12 weeks.' (Kathrin, 31)

The reasons for this are usually similar to the ones for planned freebirth.

'I didn't want the midwife sitting around while I was only 3 cm dilated, making me nervous.' (Kathrin, 31)

Some women only realise during birth that they need to be alone:

'The decision to birth alone only came during the birth though.' (Amelie, 25)

'Everyone present – never mind how nice and /or quiet – would have disturbed the process and presented a danger to my dream birth. It took a few minutes from realising that to the conclusion that I didn't want anyone, I didn't need anyone, dammit, and don't owe anyone or anything (neither people, nor societal norms).' (Magda, 26)

The transition to fully planned freebirth is smooth as well.

The planned freebirth: Celebrating your freedom and birthing power

The conscious decision to birth without a midwife present is a big step for a woman: away from societal norms towards an uninhibited 'yes' to herself and her needs and feelings. First and foremost, the need not to be disturbed and the desire for privacy contributes to the decision. Most women are sure of this.

'To surrender and to open is essential for birth. And many women, and I am one of them, do this best when they are alone or in the presence of loved and trusted ones. A freebirth, under my own steam, without outside influence, seemed the logical and honest consequence.' (Romy, 33)

'I thought, although I had no previous birth experience that I would be someone for whom maximum privacy was the most important thing during birth.' (Sandra, 41)

'Birthing is as intimate as sex or going to the toilet, and you only do that with your partner or by yourself.' (Eileen, 26)

'I find birth to be very intimate and private, like sex. I don't want anyone around who tells me what to do or is 'only' watching. I am very clear about the influence the birth attendant's feelings can have on the process! Every outside influence has to be noticed, acknowledged or ignored. This takes time and strength, disturbing the birthing woman and bringing her 'out' of herself. Any disruption or disquiet disturbs the hormonal interplay which can cause complications or simply pain.' (Sarah, 32)

Experiences from previous births, in hospital, with a midwife in the birth centre or at home, play a big role when deciding for a freebirth.

'I chose this type of birth for myself because I wanted complete freedom when it came to birth, without limitations or interventions and also because my midwife pulled the placenta from my uterus far too quickly (12 minutes after birth) during my first birth, resulting in a heavy bleed.' (Yvonne, 38)

'Because I wanted to remain whole and wished for a normal birth, finally.' (Angela, 39)

'During my first birth in the hospital, I found the examinations and monitoring with the CTG machine very disturbing. I didn't feel at home and couldn't move freely. I was limited in what I could do and felt patronised by staff.' (Birgit, 25)

'Due to my traumatic birth with my first baby (directed by others) I realised that I have to birth without intervention, otherwise my physiological birth process is disturbed.' (Lisa, 29)

Another reason is midwives feeling unable to support mothers, for example with cases of breech presentation or very overdue births.

'Due to insurance issues the midwife was not able to attend the birth with such malpositioning (breech)....she would have had to call an ambulance had I entered into a contract with her and declined transfer if she felt it appropriate. Only very few hospitals let you 'try' to birth a breech baby vaginally. A waterbirth would be contraindicated as constant CTG monitoring would be impossible, getting a woman out of the pool may be problematic and doctors don't have easy 'access'. There would be an anaesthetist and doctor present during the birth, just in case. Birthing position would either be on my back or on all fours, if I didn't have an epidural anyway. Maneuvers to deliver the arms and head would be used even during an uncomplicated birth......so my wish for a natural, unhindered birth was only possible with a freebirth!' (Stephanie, 33)

'At the end of pregnancy I went over my due date and my midwife did not want to support me anymore. She had a long chat with me and asked me to go to the hospital for a check up.' (Steffi, 28)

A woman from Australia was unable to secure the care of a midwife as homebirth had been made illegal for her specific case.

'We had just moved from Queensland, where there are lots of homebirth midwives, to the Northern Territory. Here, midwives have very strict guidelines and for example, they are not allowed to support births outside of the bigger towns. We live 3 hours by car away from Darwin and the nearest hospital, so a midwife-attended homebirth was out of the question.' (Rebekka, 33)

Women who consciously give birth without a midwife spend a lot of time informing themselves and preparing for their freebirth.

'I read a lot on the internet and read many books about complications and how to deal with them. From that I mostly learned that most risks are not actually a big deal.' (Tina, 32)

'I read lots of books on natural birth, as well as 'Unassisted Childbirth' (Shanley). In pregnancy I did lots of yoga and bellydancing and listened to lots of relaxation cds such as hypnobirthing.' (Sandra, 41)

'In my third pregnancy I wrote down exactly what is important to me during birth and how it should be. This was really helpful to guide my thoughts into that direction during the birth, so I didn't think of things I didn't want but only the things I DID want (easy and joyous birth).' (Sarah, 32)

Antenatal care

Especially the mothers who had a planned freebirth reduced traditional antenatal visits or did without them (almost) completely.

'A short doctor's visit (including two ultrasounds) until I found a midwife. Then a midwife visit without ultrasound and reduced blood tests (no HB check), but more feel good appointments for massage.' (Magda, 26)

'During the second pregnancy I went to the doctor once for an ultrasound and saw the midwife a few times, but in a very 'hands off' way, no blood tests or vaginal examinations.' (Sarah, 32)

'In my second pregnancy I only had a couple of chats with the midwife but no examinations. In my third and fourth pregnancy I had no antenatal 'care'.' (Nadine, 35)

The reasons to opt out of antenatal care are generally negative experiences in previous pregnancies and the desire to free oneself from care that is often experienced as bullying and fear mongering as well as the confidence (often only found through several pregnancies) in the woman's own trust in her intuition and power to birth her baby.

'After the birth I realised that the visits to my doctor always made me feel like I was ill despite feeling amazing and all test result being normal.' (Tina, 32)

'In my third pregnancy I finally trusted my intuition and declined antenatal care. That turned out to be the best pregnancy of all of them!' (Stefanie, 33)

'Even just the word 'Geburtshilfe' (which is the German word for obstetrics and translated literally, mean 'help to birth') makes me feel like my ability to birth is in doubt.' (Jobina, 35)

In my first pregnancy I had three chats with my local midwife. After the second one I realised that all the tests and examinations do not contribute to a healthy and joyous pregnancy and birth.' (Beatrice, 36)

Women who feel skeptical about conventional antenatal care or decline it completely usually take care of themselves very thoroughly during pregnancy. They do what makes them feel good and even find out how to get certain test results for themselves.

'I took out a lot of time, just for myself as I was conscious as to how much time I had saved by not having to go to antenatal appointments.' (Jobina, 35)

'I exercised a lot (yoga) and on the day before the birth I swam a whole kilometer.' (Caroline, 37)

'I also learned for the first time to feel for the baby's position myself.' (Stefanie, 33)

'Both pregnancies went well. No one found anything abnormal and I felt free and happy. I read a few books, watched birth DVDs and often retreated into myself. Silence is my most trusted and constant companion until today.' (Beatrice, 36)

Unusual situations and complications

Of course we asked our women about complications. These are the most common answers from the ones we received:

'I was whole, untraumatised, fit and well after all my freebirths.' (Constanze, 35)

'There were no complications.' (Saskia, 29)

'Early labour dragged on a bit as I had an Au Pair in the house and it was hard to relax. Later, the birth happened calmly, without complications. For the first time I had no problems with an anterior lip of cervix.' (Kathrin, 31)

Some of the stories contain unusual situations that would likely be classed as pathological or reason for intervention in the hospital. However, in the peace and quiet of home, those issues were (nearly) always solved or didn't present a problem in the end.

'Later when I wanted to push out the baby, progress stopped. I felt with my hand, and something was in the way. The baby had to move back up a little bit first and was then born without his hand by the side of his head.' (Tina, 32)

'After another half hour the placenta came out after our prayer. The midwife had just arrived and wanted to transfer us to hospital as the placenta was still firmly attached.' (Yvette, 32)

'The placenta came out an hour later, just before the midwife arrived.' (Saskia, 29)

'Both times my perineum tore about 6–8cm and healed by itself without problems.' (Beatrice, 36)

'We could see the place where a second placenta had been attached, and when I fished the pads out of the bin I could see the partly reabsorbed, necrotic second twin.' (Caroline, 37)

'N. was a little cold the first night. Probably because we didn't have any warm towels handy. He had a very congested face and lots of petechiae (tiny needleprick size red dots of bleeding under the skin) on his forehead and in his eyes.' (Rebekka, 26)

'She immediately turned blue and coughed. Instinctively I grabbed the cord. It was still pulsing and I felt calmed as she was still getting oxygen.' (Yvonne, 38)

'His cord was wrapped around his neck and my husband had to unwind it before he could pass him to me through my legs. I did tear a little bit but the midwife sutured the tear later without problems.' (Kathrin, 28)

'Then I felt all along her body to check if the cord was wrapped around it. It wasn't but it had torn off completely, directly at the baby's tummy! We had no cord to clamp and I put the baby on my belly to compress the wound somewhat. Then, at around 7.10am the midwife arrived and I birthed the placenta with her present. The bleeding stopped and we had to wash the baby completely.' (Lisa, 29)

Freebirth with obstacles

Nearly all planned freebirths happened as planned. But sometimes things did not go as hoped for. In one case the mother had an inkling something might not be right during the birth and called the midwife.

'At some point, I just had a weird feeling – the knowledge that I would need help. My midwife was very hands off and let me do what felt good. 1.5 hours after her arrival the baby was born with an asynclitic (tipped to the side) head – placenta after 45 minutes (no intervention) but unfortunately incomplete – manual removal by midwife.' (Sarah, 29)

In another case everything was going well but the baby was born blue and didn't breathe immediately so that the father didn't call the available midwife but an ambulance which had unnecessary dramatic consequences for mother and baby.

'My husband was unable to judge the situation appropriately and called the ambulance which caused unnecessary medical intervention. They took my son to the neonatal intensive care unit.

When I arrived there he had a gastric tube and was connected to several drips. Despite all tests being normal, they insisted on him having prophylactic antibiotics: 'When you have a homebirth, there are lots of germs about. So we are going to give these until we can prove that there is no infection.'' (Nancy, 27)

And there was one case when a caesarean was necessary to get the baby out in the end. In this case the low lying placenta detached from the uterus prematurely after membranes rupture with the baby in transverse lie:

'After my water had been broken for 32 hours without contractions I noticed that something felt different just above my symphysis pubis. The feeling was one of 'something is rummaging around in my belly' and later turned into discomfort. I went to the toilet because I thought I might be losing more liquor (which gets produced constantly, the baby was not 'dry' for 32 hours). This is where I noticed that I was not losing liquor but blood. The bleeding was like a constant thin stream of water. I tried to get dressed but all pads and clothes immediately got soaked so I called the hospital to tell them that I needed to come in, told them my history as well as informing them that I would need an emergency section and to please get theatre ready. The grandparents were already with the older children and took me and my husband to the hospital. There I was in theatre very quickly, shortly after a vaginal examination. 30 minutes after the bleeding started our baby was born, with collapsed umbilical cord and the need for resuscitation. (Severe asphyxia, Apgars 3/4/6). Immediately before the section the baby had turned back into transverse lie.' (Seraphine, 41)

Small and still freebirths

Even when a baby doesn't survive in the womb for some reason, some women would rather deal with this situation without medical intervention. These women trust their bodies to be able to manage birthing these small or still babies without outside help. The reasons for an unattended miscarriage or stillbirth are the same in principle as for freebirth with a live child.

Annalies experienced a miscarriage by herself in the 13th week of pregnancy:

'When I was told (by her midwife, author) that complications would be unlikely as long as I felt healthy and the risk of infection would be similar to after a D&C in the hospital, it was clear to me that I wanted to let nature take its course.' (Annalies, 39)

Katharina (28) had an unattended 'small birth' in the 10th week of pregnancy:

'I didn't want to go back to the hospital to have an operation. I already had a D&C after my second birth. I felt that I needed to and could do this by myself. No one could really help me anyway and I could call for help, should it become necessary.'

Rarely the baby's life ends later in pregnancy. Kerstin tells of her self-directed stillbirth in the 27th week of pregnancy:

'I wanted the security of my own home, and to be able to enjoy the few moments I had with my baby who had already died in utero in peace, without any medical intervention or direction, in full awareness.'

Anna (25) went to hospital in early pregnancy but didn't want to stay there:

'In hospital they told me that my baby was still alive, the heart was beating but that I would lose the baby soon. I didn't want to stay there under any circumstances and drove home.'

It is not rare that several weeks pass between diagnosis of the baby's death and the actual miscarriage:

'I felt the loss and grieved. Interestingly I got the time for that because saying goodbye took about 4 weeks. My midwife gave me advice about what I could do for worries and heavy bleeding with herbal teas and homeopathy. Then came the waiting and observing how my body very slowly turned 'unpregnant'. I could practically feel how my pregnancy hormone levels dropped and the

end of pregnancy got closer and closer.' (Annalies, 39)

Despite the sadness that comes with birthing a baby that has passed away in utero, the experience of doing so in a self-directed way while trusting her body can give women strength and confidence for subsequent pregnancies.

Annalies (39) reports:

'After the miscarriage I rested in bed for a about a day, reflecting on the experience and – this might sound odd, but – happy. I had managed by myself. All in all a very healing experience … In my third pregnancy, this experience turned out to be my anchor. I had the feeling all would be well if I could make my own decisions.'

The mothers in this book

On the following pages we will hear from the mothers who were happy to become part of this book in their own words and pictures.

The page layout will always follow the same format.

On the left of the page you will find a short introduction of the mother, including:

- Mother's first name (some mothers have changed their names to maintain anonymity)
- Age at the time of interview
- Job title
- Children, with sex, age and type of birth respectively

On the top right on every left hand page you will also find a quote from the interview.

The interview follows, in the mother's actual words, but some may have been shortened by the author with the mother's consent.

On the right hand side are photos to give you an insight into the families. They have been taken from the families' personal collections. In three cases (Sarah, 32; Stefanie, 33; Annalies, 39) the interview stretches over 4 pages.

The reports, planned, unplanned and half planned freebirths, have been sorted by age of participant and if the age was identical, by alphabetical order. As the transition from planned, half planned and unplanned freebirth is so fluid and some participants had an unplanned or half planned freebirth first and then a planned one, there was no further categorisation.

Unplanned and half planned freebirths are marked as such, but planned freebirths are only headed as 'freebirth'.

Following that, also sorted alphabetically, you can find the chapter on freebirths with obstacles and after that, small and still freebirths.

Some numbers

Between January and March 2014 we recruited 36 women who were happy to talk about their freebirth experiences with us for our project.

Our youngest participant is 25 and our oldest 48, the average age is 33.1 years old.

The vast majority of participants, 27 of them, are from Germany. Following are women from Switzerland. Then one each from Austria, Spain and Australia.

Altogether the women in this book have given birth to 103 children, including one set of twins. On average each woman had 3.0 children, well over the German average of 1.38 (German Federal Office of Statistics 2012).

44 of those children were born without a midwife present. Two births planned as freebirth didn't happen as such. Additionally we have five reports of small birth (two by the same woman) and one stillbirth. Each mother talks about at least one and at most three freebirths. Some women who talk about their freebirths also mention a small freebirth in their story. But because the focus in those cases is on the life freebirth we have only mentioned the miscarriage when the participant wrote about it and wanted us to.

Of the rest of the children, 30 were born in hospital, 19 in a birth centre and 10 at home attended by a midwife.

Four women share their experience of caesarean birth in their story. Another four women who were pregnant again at the time of the interview all planned another freebirth or at least kept open the option of calling the midwife too late.

Unplanned, half planned
and planned freebirths

Amelie, 25
Job title: Photographer

**"I dreamt of birthing my baby
by myself during the night."**

1st Child: Girl (4y), hospital birth
2nd Child: Girl (5mo), half planned freebirth

When I hear the word 'freebirth', the following thoughts pop into my head: Maximum self-determination, calm, no interruptions.

When did you first have the idea to birth without a midwife? Sometime in the middle of pregnancy. The decision to birth alone only came during the birth though.

Who did you tell of your plans? I told my friend (who also had homebirths) that I dreamt of having the baby by myself during the night. Her reaction was shock: 'Please don't do that! What if something goes wrong?' I also told my second midwife, who I saw for a foot massage a few times during pregnancy, about my dream and asked what her take on freebirth was. She said she was generally not opposed but thought I was not quite in the right place for it yet, maybe in my third pregnancy.

How did the pregnancy go and who did your antenatal care? Lovely. I felt good from the beginning and had a good bond with my baby. We – my husband, my daughter and I – we were looking forward to the little one.

I already contacted my midwife in my 7th week of pregnancy as I knew it would be difficult to find a homebirth midwife later on. I liked her immediately and decided to let her do all my antenatal care apart from a second trimester ultrasound.

Compared to my first pregnancy in which I had seen a doctor exclusively I found midwifery care a total luxury.

Why did you choose freebirth for yourself? Because it was the best thing at the time. I'm not sure I could have stayed as relaxed with the

midwife present, possibly giving me instructions. Yes, even talking would have disturbed me. My husband and I only exchanged a few quiet words during the breaks between contractions.

How did you prepare for the birth? I bought the book 'Hypnobirthing' at the beginning of my pregnancy, which became my companion for the remainder of my pregnancy. The book gave me a lot of confidence and knowledge, for example about how the muscles of the uterus work together. I found the relaxation exercises easy. I did them every night and listened to the relaxation tracks.

How did the birth go – any complications? The birth started on the sixth day after my due date. It was a lovely warm day and my husband, daughter and I went for a long walk in the early evening to get the first surges going.

Around 20.30 I put my daughter to bed and breastfed her for an extra long time to get her to sleep, which made the surges stronger. Around 21.30 I went on a second walk, alone this time. I was in a good mood, enjoyed the warm air and talked to my baby about how lovely it would be for her to be born.

I kept looking at my phone to keep an eye on the contractions. They came every 3 minutes by now and I went back home. The surges were pleasant and I was using the slow breathing I had learned from the hypnobirthing book during my pregnancy.

When I arrived home I told my husband that things would start soon and went to bed where I slept for about an hour. Around one o'clock I got back up as the surges had intensified. I decided to have a bath. I felt good and was completely relaxed.

My husband came into the bathroom and asked if we should call the midwife or the friends we had planned to have present. Until then I hadn't even thought of that! I said that we should wait a bit.

During a break in contractions I suddenly felt the need to go to the loo where my waters went and the surges became even more intense but not painful. My husband asked again if he should call the midwife and I declined yet again.

I went onto all fours for the next contraction. I had very strong pressure downwards. With one hand I protected my perineum and could already feel the baby's head.

Then we heard my older daughter wake up. My husband got her and put her next to me. At first she was a little confused but I calmed her down quickly and told her that everything was ok and our baby was being born now. I used the breathing method I had learned in pregnancy and could feel how my body and my baby worked together, all by themselves.

I didn't push, only breathed deeply and suddenly I felt the whole head in my hand. The body followed a few seconds later, around 1.35am, and I held my baby in my arms.

'That was so easy. That was so easy' I exclaimed again and again. My husband had called the midwife a few minutes before the birth so she arrived about 15 minutes after when we were already snuggled in bed.

How did you experience the postnatal period? I hardly left my bed in the first few days. My husband looked after the older child, sorted the household and cooked for me. We only allowed visitors in small doses, our parents briefly popped by on the first day and selected family and friends on the following days. It was a lovely time, except for the third day which was difficult as I was struggling with blocked ducts and retained lochia. My midwife was of great help, she came to visit us daily in the first week and I always looked forward to her visits.

What would you tell other mothers-to-be? Listen to your heart and your intuition! In your pregnancy, surround yourself with people that make you feel good and enjoy the precious time.

What would you do differently during another pregnancy and birth? I don't think I would do anything differently. For us, this was the right way, the birth was beautiful, pain free and self-directed.

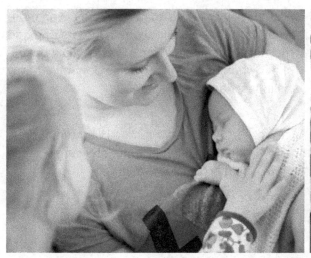
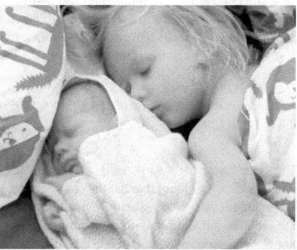

Self-Directed Pregnancy and Birth

Birgit, 25
Job Title: Mother and Homemaker

1st Child: Boy (7 y), hospital birth
2nd Child: Girl (1 y), freebirth

"Nobody to tell me what to do and make decisions for me."

When I hear the word 'freebirth', the following thoughts pop into my head: A woman can birth in a self-directed way. No disrupting exams. I can move freely and do what feels good. A gentle start in life for a newborn. Nobody to tell me what to do and make decisions for me.

When did you first have the idea to birth without a midwife? At the beginning of my second pregnancy ...

Who did you tell of your plans? Everyone who asked where I would have my baby. I saw no reason to lie just to avoid discussion.

How did the pregnancy go and who did your antenatal care? I had no complications during pregnancy and only went to the doctor 3 times. I declined all further care.

Why did you choose freebirth for yourself? Birth is something very intimate to me and I didn't want to put up with strangers around me. During my first birth in the hospital I found the constant checks and CTG monitoring very disrupting. I didn't feel at home and wasn't able to move around freely. I was very limited in what I could do and felt patronised by the hospital staff.

How did you prepare for the birth? I had a chat with a midwife, and joined a group on the internet.

How did the birth go – any complications? The birth was calm and relaxed. I walked a lot and was busy breathing through the contractions. When labour was already very advanced, my legs felt really numb and I had no choice but to sit or kneel. I screamed a lot, loudly, into a pillow. It felt really relaxing and I felt like it really made the birth move forward. After midnight I felt strong pressure and started pushing. I went onto my knees and lent on the sofa. After few minutes the head was born and my partner sat behind me to receive the baby. Then we woke the big brother to say hello to the new arrival. After an hour our older child was allowed to cut the cord with his father's help. The placenta came a couple of hours later.

At first I put our daughter to the breast to stimulate the uterus to contract down. The bleeding did not stop however. I pushed on my uterus via my belly – but that didn't help either. I asked our son to get a towel soaked in cold water that I then put on my belly. A few minutes later, the bleeding reduced. Even this unusual situation was dealt with calmly and without panic.

How did you experience the postnatal period? Oh, it was really lovely. All of us spent a lot of time snuggling in our big family bed and had plenty of time to get to know each other.

What would you tell other mothers-to-be? It is amazing to get to know your body even more during birth. We have to learn to understand and trust ourselves again. A birth is something beautiful but when it happens in a self determined way it is indescribably amazing.

What would you do differently during another pregnancy and birth? In a normal pregnancy I would decline any antenatal care. For the birth I would do the same again.

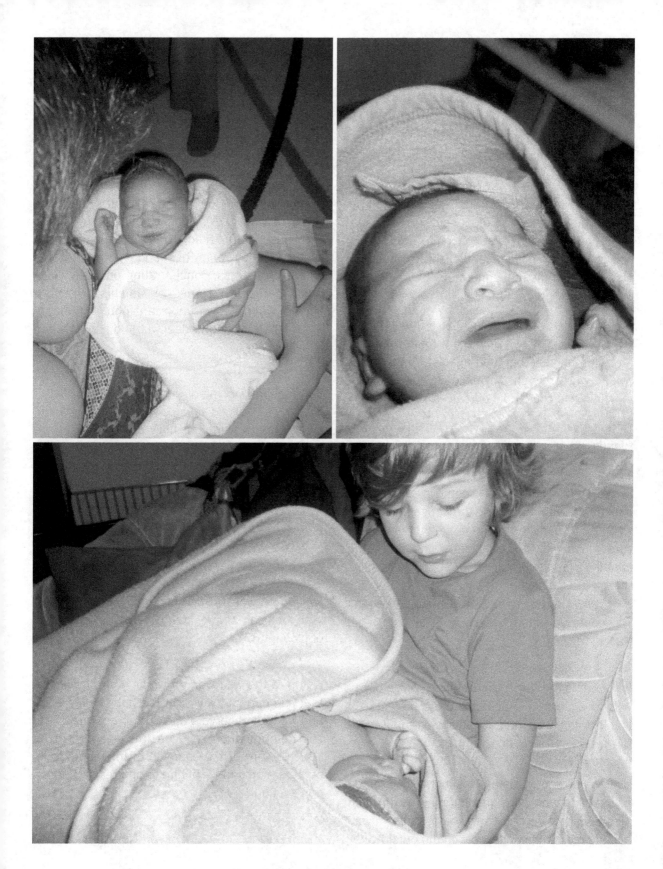

Self-Directed Pregnancy and Birth

Eileen, 26
Job Title: Teacher

1st Child: Girl (6 y), hospital birth
2nd Child: Girl (3 y), birth center birth
3rd Child: Boy (9 mo), freebirth

"After 5 hours I birthed our sunny side up baby kneeling, in the water, no pushing, no tears."

When I hear the word 'freebirth', the following thoughts pop into my head: Self-determination, power, full responsibility, I can surrender completely and let go, comfort for mother and child, trust in God, candlelight, my husband playing guitar, the most enormous and empowering experience of my life.

When did you first have the idea to birth without a midwife? Before my third pregnancy. My common sense argued against it initially but when I was pregnant, my child gave me impulse to believe we could do it ourselves.

Who did you tell of your plans? Family and friends.

How did the pregnancy go and who did your antenatal care? No complications but exhausting due to renovating the house and severe sickness towards the end of pregnancy. Antenatal care from a midwife (no vaginal examinations, etc, chatting was important to me, especially about the spiritual aspect of my pregnancy). I never saw a doctor and didn't want any ultrasound scans. The communication between me and my child was strong.

Why did you choose freebirth for yourself? Freebirth is the safest and gentlest way to birth a baby. It ensures a peaceful and dignified start in life. Birthing is as intimate as sex or going to the toilet, and you only do that with your partner or by yourself.

Midwife or doctor disturb instinct and intuition, even well meaning tips are disruptive as the woman's body know what it has to do. I trust myself and life more than an 'expert on the outside'.

How did you prepare for the birth? By reading, for example: 'Unassisted Childbirth' (Shanley), Babyglück (Wenger), Gebären ohne Aberglauben (Rockenschaub) – meditation – creating my birth space – chats with my husband – going for walks – reducing stress, concentrating on positives – reading freebirth stories or watching freebirth films – writing down important phone numbers – refreshed my knowledge: what do I do if I bleed heavily? First Aid?

How did the birth go – any complications? Contractions started during the night. We lit candles and I vocalised 'oooooooh' and 'aaaaaaaaah' loudly in the warm birthing pool. Contractions were very painful this time, but everything was beautiful. After 5 hours I birthed our sunny side up baby kneeling, in the water, no pushing, no tears. The baby's sisters woke shortly after and were amazed.

How did you experience the postnatal period? Like a queen, deeply peaceful and in endless love. I snuggled my baby in the bedroom for two whole weeks, my husband, parents and in laws took care of me. I felt powerful (I ate a piece of placenta).

What would you tell other mothers-to-be? Listen to the wild woman within you. She knows that she can and will birth the baby in seclusion and without observers and authority figures, with self determination. YOU are the only expert on YOU! Beware of the cascade of intervention: Induction – epidural – failure to progress – Caesarean section!

What would you do differently during another pregnancy and birth? Nothing!

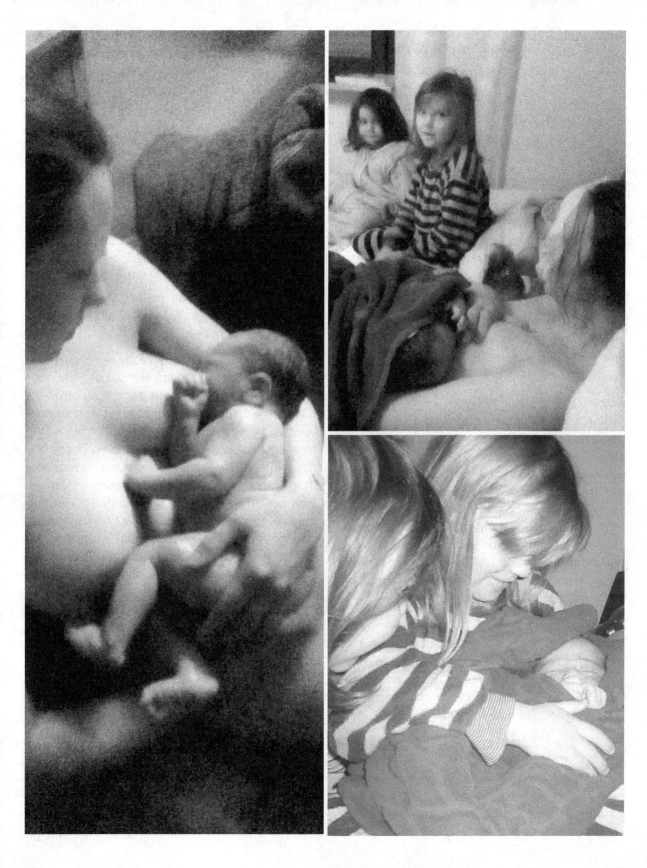

Magda, 26
Job Title: Educator (BA, self employed in parent education)

1st Child: Girl (9 y), hospital birth
2nd Child: Boy (4 y), half planned freebirth
3rd Child: Boy (1.5 y) freebirth

"The realisation that I didn't need or want anyone there only came when contractions had already started."

When I hear the word 'freebirth', the following thoughts pop into my head: Self determination. Safety from intervention, only real option to birth a baby, primal elemental forces. A birth experience such as this is every woman's and child's birth right!

When did you first have the idea to birth without a midwife? In my second pregnancy, on my journey from hospital to home birth. It was more a flirting with the idea rather than a concrete plan.

Who did you tell of your plans? No one, because the decision for a freebirth only really happened during the birth. The realisation that I didn't need or want anyone there only came when contractions had already started. Before the second freebirth it was clear I would do the same again. Everyone who was interested knew, including the midwife doing my antenatal care. The implicitness of my decision and my wide knowledge regarding all 'What if....?' questions stopped all negative comments etc. in their tracks or from being brought up in the first place.

How did the pregnancy go and who did your antenatal care? A short doctor's visit (including two ultrasounds) until I found a midwife. Then a midwife visit without ultrasound and reduced bloodtests (no HB check), but more 'feel good' appointments for massage.

Why did you choose freebirth for yourself? The first freebirth was more of a spontaneous idea. Thanks to good information and being in tune with my body I realised that I didn't want anyone present and more importantly didn't need anyone. Everyone present – never mind how nice

and/or quiet – would have disturbed the process and presented a danger to my dream birth. It took a few minutes from realising that to the conclusion that I didn't want anyone, I didn't need anyone, dammit, and don't owe anyone or anything (neither people, nor societal norms).

My second freebirth was the logical consequence of the previous incredibly enriching and empowering birth experience.

Since I found out how birth really works (Just like that! Under my own steam, without disturbance/ observation or intervention) there is no other option for me anymore. Freebirth is the only guarantee that no one will ask something at the wrong moment, suggest something or even check you (for example the baby's heartbeat) to reassure themselves. Even a certain look can turn an amazingly powerful experience into horrific torture. You only get to do this birth once! For my own safety and that of my child I need to make sure that the birth can proceed optimally. And that is only possible when I have eliminated the unpredictability that comes from other people.

How did you prepare for the birth? I read, read and read some more. Mostly, good specialist literature. How does birth work? What can go wrong and why? How can I prevent complications and what do I do when I encounter them anyway? Obstetrical knowledge in combination with my instinct for my baby's well being and my own body gives me more wisdom (and security) than any outsider ever could.

How did the birth go – ny complications?
1. Freebirth 4 hours. Uncomplicated, powerful, nearly pain free with a long and exhausting

second stage. The sheer power and primal force were sometimes hard to cope with. 2. Freebirth: Started with waters breaking. Slight first stage contractions, short transitional phase, then only 3 pushing contractions. Pain free as well as uncomplicated.

How did you experience the postnatal period? The postnatal period was tainted by external trouble (moving house) and lots of chaos. Despite this, my baby was as relaxed in the early days as the birth was easy.

What would you tell other mothers-to-be? Read lots and have more trust in yourself and your baby and less in the 'experts'. No one can know your body better than yourself!

Large parts of antenatal 'care' and obstetrics serve to reassure doctors and midwives and don't assure the health of mother and baby. We are service users in hospitals, when going to the doctor or while having any other type of medical care. WE decide. Nobody can decide for us or the baby, allow or disallow us or tell us what to do. Suggestions yes, regulations no. Have courage for open dialogue and to use the word: 'No!'

What would you do differently during another pregnancy and birth? Not much. Perhaps I would have more appointments for things like massage or other holistic therapies to pamper myself and to dedicate more time to the unborn and the pregnancy.

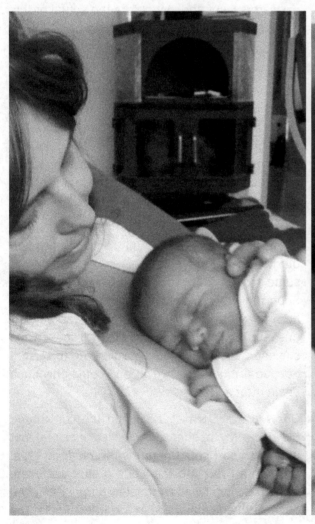 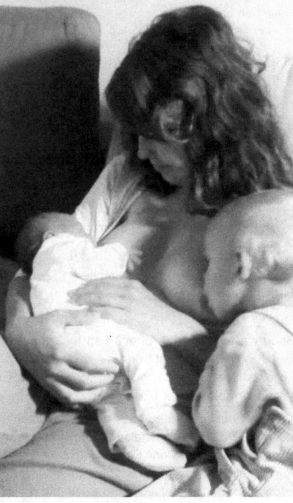

Self-Directed Pregnancy and Birth

Rebekka, 26
Job Title: Homemaker and mother

"Our baby wasn't as light and small as expected. Everything happened quickly anyway!"

1st Child: Boy (5 y), hospital birth
2nd Child: Girl (3 y), homebirth
3rd Child: Boy (5 mo), unplanned freebirth/planned homebirth

When I hear the word 'freebirth', the following thoughts pop into my head: Undisturbed, self determined birth.

When did you first have the idea to birth without a midwife? We didn't actually plan a freebirth but another homebirth with our midwife. I had thought about it in my third pregnancy because the first two births happened quickly, the midwife didn't have any back up and the hospital wasn't an option for us.

Who did you tell of your plans? My husband and I talked about it a few times. Apart from that, nobody.

How did the pregnancy go and who did your antenatal care? The pregnancy went by without any complications or complaints. My midwife did the antenatal care and I went to the doctor twice for ultrasounds.

Why did you choose freebirth for yourself? It just turned out like that and wasn't planned.

How did you prepare for the birth? I had read a few birth stories and watched a few freebirth videos.

How did the birth go – any complications? Shortly after midnight, after I had just gone to bed, I could feel the first twinges in my lower belly. Followed by another, and another. Lying down was uncomfortable so I got back up.

I told my husband to go back to sleep, I wasn't quite sure if this was a false alarm or the real thing. I had not had any Braxton Hicks contractions the whole pregnancy. The twinges came every 2-3 minutes, I felt good by myself and could breathe the contractions away. I woke my husband again at around 1.20. I was sure that our baby would be born that night and wanted him there in case I needed him.

We had a quick chat and then I noticed that I needed the toilet urgently. This is when I noticed I was bleeding and felt a bit unsettled. During the first two births this only happened shortly after my waters went and just before the actual births. But I didn't feel I was at that point yet.

I asked my husband to call the midwife. At 1.36 he got through to her and asked me if she should come yet as it seemed a little early in the process. She didn't wait for my answer but said she'd be on her way. She thought the baby was rather small and light and it could all happen very quickly. While my husband started to prep the living room, I wanted to check my cervix and see how far open it was. To my surprise I only felt the baby's head quite low down in my vagina.

My husband tried to help me to the living room but I could not move anymore so he brought me some towels to kneel on and sat behind me. Soon my waters went and the baby's head was born straight after. When the head was out, my husband got nervous. He thought it looked too squished and too blue and asked me to push. I needed a moment however and could only push again after a little break.

Our son was born at 1.50 with the cord round his neck. My husband unravelled him and put him down so I could bring him through my legs. Our son arrived into the world a little confused, without crying. I was completely surprised by the quick birth and marvelled at our little miracle. The placenta was born soon after and some minutes later our midwife arrived. Weighing 3740g and 50cm long, our baby wasn't as light and small as expected. Everything happened quickly anyway!

He was a little cold during the first night. Probably because we didn't have any warm towels handy. He had a very congested face and lots of petechiae (tiny needleprick sized red dots of bleeding under the skin) on his forehead and in his eyes, either because of the cord round his neck or because he got a little stuck at some point.

How did you experience the postnatal period? I was very well, no tears and nearly no afterpains. It was a shame that my husband had to go back to work full time on the fourth day after the birth. I didn't want strangers in my house and no family members could make it so I had to get on with things by myself. I would have liked to have more time to just snuggle the baby and do nothing else.

What would you tell other mothers-to-be? Trust your body.

What would you do differently during another pregnancy and birth? I would like less antenatal care. My midwife wanted to test for lots of things this pregnancy. And I would like to be by myself for longer after the birth. Although on the one hand I was glad my midwife came after the birth, on the other hand I found it quite disruptive.

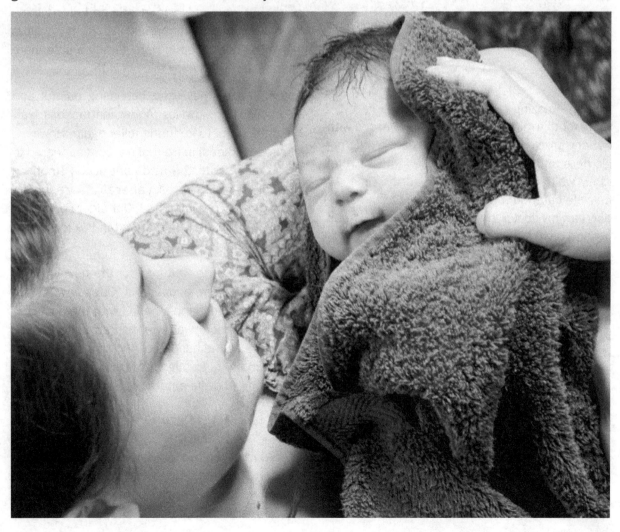

Kathrin, 28
Job Title: Student

"Listen to your gut and allow any thoughts at all, even the outlandish ones."

1st Child: Boy (4 y), homebirth
2nd Child: Boy (5 mo), unplanned freebirth/planned homebirth

When I hear the word 'freebirth', the following thoughts pop into my head: Self confidence, comfort, rising above yourself.

When did you first have the idea to birth without a midwife? Subconsciously I have always been drawn towards it. But I didn't really allow the thought. I planned the birth with my husband, my son and my midwife.

Who did you tell of your plans? Nobody, not even myself, really.

How did the pregnancy go and who did your antenatal care? The pregnancy for us was an amazing present. We had waited 1 1/2 years for this miracle. The pregnancy passed without any problems as my first one had. A little niggle here and there, but otherwise fantastic. I felt really well and very much enjoyed the time. My midwife cared for me from the start to the end. I only saw my doctor three times for routine screening and once for unexplained pain in my cervix.

Why did you choose freebirth for yourself? I didn't choose it consciously. I did tinker with the thought and quietly admired the women who did, but I didn't consider it for myself. I assumed I couldn't manage it and therefore didn't go down that route.

How did you prepare for the birth? I read lots of out of hospital birth stories and viewed lots of birth videos on the internet. I sort of knew what was coming from my previous birth. It was important to me to properly prepare for the inevitable end of pregnancy. I really struggled with the end of the lovely time of pregnancy after my first birth and wanted to preempt it this time.

How did the birth go – any complications? The birth began on the day I absolutely didn't want it to start – Christmas Eve. I already had a funny feeling during the night before but decided it was just me feeling tense because labour wasn't allowed to start in the next few days. I had my show that morning.

Contractions came every 3-4 minutes at that point, but were only very gentle so I didn't think birth was imminent. Around 11.25 my waters went. The contractions were getting a little more intense, but were easy to cope with.

Around 12.10 they were becoming painful and we called the midwives. A few contractions later I had the need to go to the toilet again. However, the need to kneel in front of the sofa appeared to be stronger. With the next contraction I noticed that I didn't need the toilet after all ... my husband could already see the head. Our older son joined us, he had up until then stayed in the room next door.

We didn't have to wait long for the next contraction and the head popped out. Our son was born fully into my husband's hands with the next contraction. His cord was wrapped around his neck and my husband had to unwind it before he could pass him to me through my legs. I did tear a little bit but the midwife sutured the tear later without problems

How did you experience the postnatal period? I really enjoyed it. However, it was cut rather short. I felt tense and found it difficult not to be able to give as much attention as I wanted to my older son. I also found it difficult watching my husband manage the household. He really really tried hard, but no one can do it right for me :-)

What would you tell other mothers-to-be? Listen to your gut and allow any thoughts at all, even the outlandish ones. It is your birth and it is unique. This is why you should do exactly what you want. It will make you stronger and you can benefit from that in your weaker moments.

What would you do differently during another pregnancy and birth? I don't think I would do anything differently. Of course I would try to enjoy the time more, but otherwise, everything felt right the way it was.

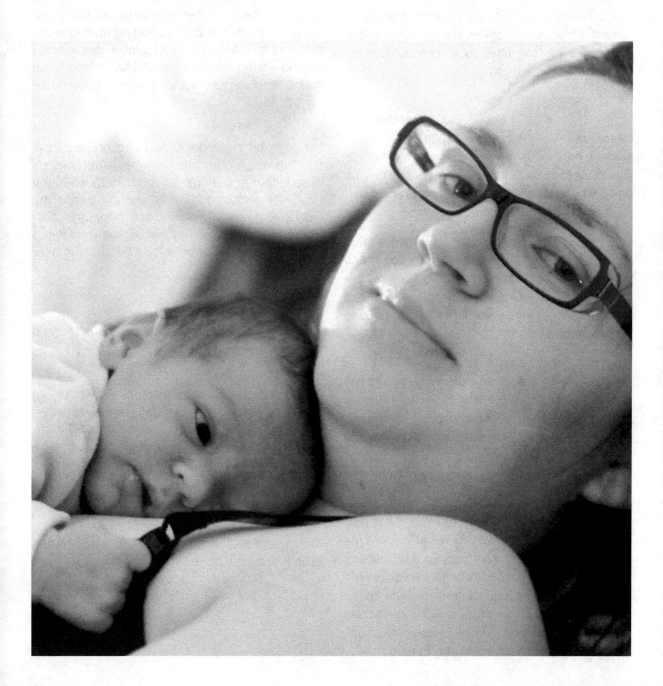

Steffi, 28
Job Title: Student

1st Child: Girl (4 y), homebirth
2nd Child: Girl (1 y), half planned freebirth

"At the end of pregnancy I went over my due date and my midwife did not want to support me anymore."

When I hear the word 'freebirth', the following thoughts pop into my head: Wonderful, vibrant, empowering, power, the most incredible experience you can have as a woman, unconditional love, beautiful pain.

When did you first have the idea to birth without a midwife? I already did during the pregnancy with my first child, but then again in the second pregnancy, partly because my midwife was going to be away at the end of my due month, and partly because I went overdue and she didn't want to support me anymore.

Who did you tell of your plans? My husband, 2-3 friends and, in great detail, a good friend who was going to support me during the freebirth (to potentially drive me to the hospital 7 minutes away in case of problems, so I wouldn't have to call an ambulance)

How did the pregnancy go and who did your antenatal care? Problem free pregnancy with some nausea. Antenatal care was provided by my doctor, later a different doctor and my midwife. At the end of pregnancy a friend (who is a doula) came to visit.

Why did you choose freebirth for yourself? At the end of pregnancy I went over my due date and my midwife did not want to support me anymore. She had a long chat with me and asked me to go to the hospital for a check up. My husband and I went to one of the hospitals and realised that I would not be able to birth my baby there. On the morning of the birth, which was the day after the hospital visit, I knew I was having 'real' contractions and that I would stay at home.

How did you prepare for the birth? I had sorted all the stuff the homebirth midwife wanted, so I just left it at that. I also told my friend but that was it. Thanks to our first lovely homebirth I had no worries for the second. I had a wonderful midwife from Ingolstadt as a phone back up by my side too.

How did the birth go – any complications? Very relaxed and wonderful. I had prepared the bathtub and during the last expulsive contractions I stood up. Things stopped briefly when the head was almost out but I somehow turned the baby slightly myself and she just 'flopped' out after. She looked at me with her big eyes and didn't cry – it was simply unbelievably relaxed and wonderful.

How did you experience the postnatal period? Not intensively, I lay on the sofa and in bed sometimes but because I also had the older child I was up most of the time.

What would you tell other mothers-to-be? Listen to your gut, your physiology – I didn't want a hospital birth because I didn't want anyone else deciding for me and no one else's hands on my baby after birth!!! A hospital is great when there are problems, and I would have transferred in that case. For everyone who is healthy, home (or wherever you feel at home) is ideal.

What would you do differently during another pregnancy and birth? To trust myself even more. Less doubt.

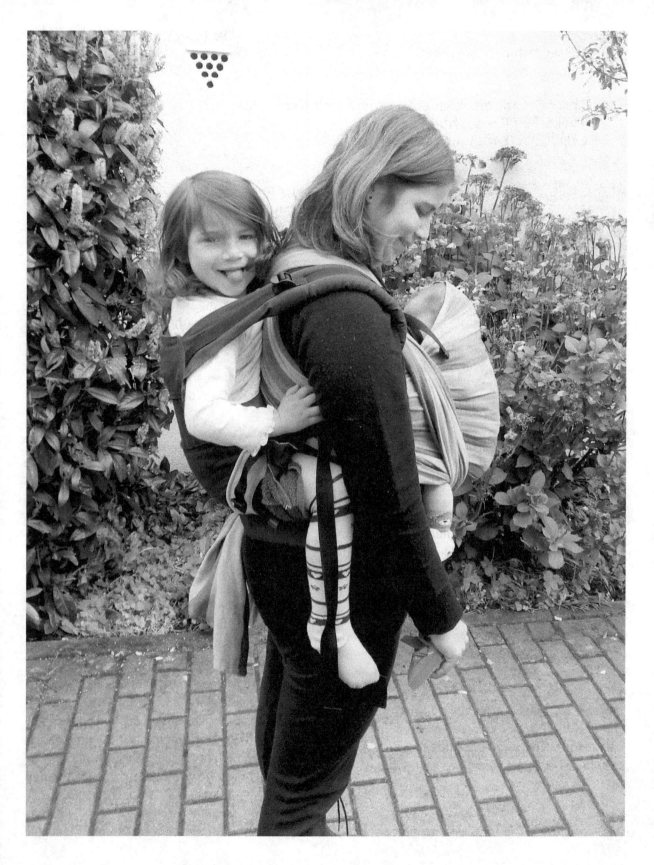

Self-Directed Pregnancy and Birth

Lisa, 29
Job Title: Anthroposophical nurse

"So I decided to do it like that anyway as I alone am responsible for me and my baby."

1st Child: Girl (nearly 4 y), birth center birth (Ventouse)
2nd Child: Boy (2.5 y), homebirth
3rd Child: Girl (8 mo), unplanned freebirth

When I hear the word 'freebirth', the following thoughts pop into my head: Calm, being myself, retreat into myself, self confidence, unhindered, natural course. And of course you are never alone during a birth (as Alleingeburt, the German word for freebirth might imply), there are always two people involved. Also, the inner bond with the child.

When did you first have the idea to birth without a midwife? I had the idea in my third pregnancy. But I thought I'd want some support, at least in the next room. So I was definitely going to have a midwife ...

The fact that everything went so well without a midwife gives me a great feeling of security with regards to a potential further birth.

Who did you tell of your plans? Everyone knew about the planned homebirth. Reactions were entirely positive. I only spoke about freebirth a few times with my friend who was also pregnant at the time.

How did the pregnancy go and who did your antenatal care? This pregnancy was entirely uncomplicated again, yet more exhausting as I have two toddlers to look after now. Several different midwives did my antenatal care. My original one got pregnant herself so I had to find a new one, but it actually worked out well. I went to the doctor once for routine screening and to the hospital for monitoring once as an emergency in later pregnancy.

Why did you choose freebirth for yourself? Due to my traumatic birth with my first baby (directed by others) I realised that I have to birth without intervention, otherwise my physiological birth process is disturbed. My second baby was born with midwives who very much stayed in the background.

I wanted the same again for my third birth. Unfortunately my midwife acted almost insulted when I asked if I could call her at the latest possible moment so nobody would disturb my labour. So I decided to do it like that anyway as I alone am responsible for me and my baby. But it happened slightly differently in the end ...

How did you prepare for the birth? I did yoga for pregnancy again, chatted lots with midwives and met up with a pregnant friend. I also saw an osteopath three times due to a twisted lumbar spine. She suspected that this played a role in my last two lengthy and difficult births. I also tried to stay as mobile as possible to make labour easier on my body.

How did the birth go – any complications? When I woke on the 24/5 (40+1) at 4.20am, I soon realised that I was having proper labour contractions (I had been having niggles now and then since seeing the osteopath 10 days earlier).

I decided to go back to bed and rest as I was expecting labour to last the whole day. I couldn't stay there for long though. Soon I could not lay down anymore due to the strength of the contractions and I woke my husband. At 6am we decided to call the midwife who was due to go on a study day that day. She advised me to call her colleague at around 8am who was her back up (she was the midwife who was there at the birth of my second baby). We went into the living room where I was leaning on different items of furniture and ate a sandwich between contractions. Around 6.15 I thought: 'If it carries on like this I won't be able to cope all day.' so I called the midwife. She heard me vocalise through a contraction and said she was coming straight away (40 minutes drive away).

I had to fully concentrate on the contractions now and hung on to my husband. Suddenly I could feel my amniotic sac bulge like a balloon. It popped with the first expulsive contraction. When I put my hand down I could already feel the head!

My husband quickly pulled my trousers down and I pushed really gently to stop my perineum from tearing. And then she shot out completely (it was 6.37am)! I had thought about squatting when the head was born ... my husband quickly picked her up and I had the strong feeling that she had to start breathing right away, so I rubbed her back.

Then I felt all along her body to check if the cord was wrapped around it. It wasn't but it had torn off completely, directly at the baby's tummy! We had no cord to clamp and I put the baby on my belly to compress the wound somewhat. Then, at around 7.10am the midwife arrived and I birthed the placenta with her present. The bleeding stopped and we had to wash the baby completely. A girl was born, a really precipitate birth, but completely healthy.

How did you experience the postnatal period? We quickly slipped back into everyday life because I felt fine. The afterpains were worse than the whole birth however, despite me eating a piece of placenta.

What would you tell other mothers-to-be? You are strong, in your unique way! You move in the stream of women that has been flowing for millenia. What energy! Feel free, untethered and grounded, be yourself during birth (and sing!). This is how things will take their natural course.

What would you do differently during another pregnancy and birth? Nothing, as nothing happens as planned, because every baby is different.

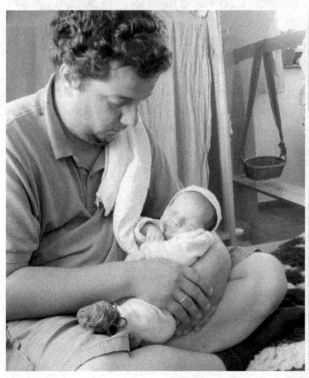
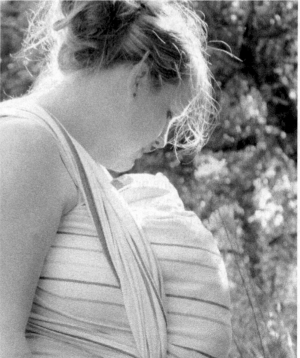

Saskia, 29
Beruf: Job Title: Dental technician,
   on maternity leave

"When I decided to just follow my body and push it was clear my midwife wouldn't make it in time."

1st Child: Boy (5 y), hospital birth with independent midwife
2nd Child: Girl (3 y), hospital birth with independent midwife
3rd Child: Girl (8 mo), unplanned freebirth

When I hear the word 'freebirth', the following thoughts pop into my head: Calm, being myself, no unnecessary and dangerous interventions, primal forces.

When did you first have the idea to birth without a midwife? Even before the pregnancy with our third child. When I realised how lucky me and my children were that the first two births happened without complications despite interventions. When I understood how pathologically minded the field of modern obstetrics is.

Who did you tell of your plans? My husband and later my midwife.

How did the pregnancy go and who did your antenatal care? The pregnancy was unremarkable, I had sporadic episodes of antenatal care, when I felt the need to, from my homebirth midwife. I also had 2 scans to exclude any major abnormalities in the 14th and 22nd week of pregnancy by the local doctor, with the caveat not to look for the baby's sex.

Why did you choose freebirth for yourself? I kept the option of freebirth open for myself as I wanted to decide spontaneously by gut feeling if I should call my midwife or not. During the birth I was very sure that everything was fine. During transition though I felt like I did want my midwife as I was unable to feel my cervix and wanted her to check it was completely open. When I decided to just follow my body and push it was clear my midwife wouldn't make it in time. I didn't have any fears and was very assured and felt safe.

How did you prepare for the birth? I ate well, was very active, read a lot about physiological birth and management of emergencies and trusted my intuition.

How did the birth go – any complications? The birth was nearly without stress. I mobilised a lot, didn't need to go anywhere and concentrated on myself. My husband kept topping up the pool with hot water, massaged my back and radiated calm with his presence. I waited for a long time for the urge to push which never came. I didn't know what my cervix was doing but then decided by gut feeling to just push anyway and shortly after my daughter swam into my hands. There were no complications. The placenta came an hour later, just before my midwife arrived. I doubt the hospital staff would have left the placenta in situ for a whole hour.

How did you experience the postnatal period? I was at home straight away, we were a family immediately, together with the older siblings. It was absolutely wonderful to just get into my own bed with the little one. I was and am so proud of this birth. My husband and I have birthed this baby all by ourselves.

What would you tell other mothers-to-be? Get informed, be clear about what is important for you and fight for it. Understand how birth works. Have courage to walk an alternative path, think outside the box. Don't blindly accept what society expects.

What would you do differently during another pregnancy and birth? I would not have an ultrasound scan in the 14th week of pregnancy.

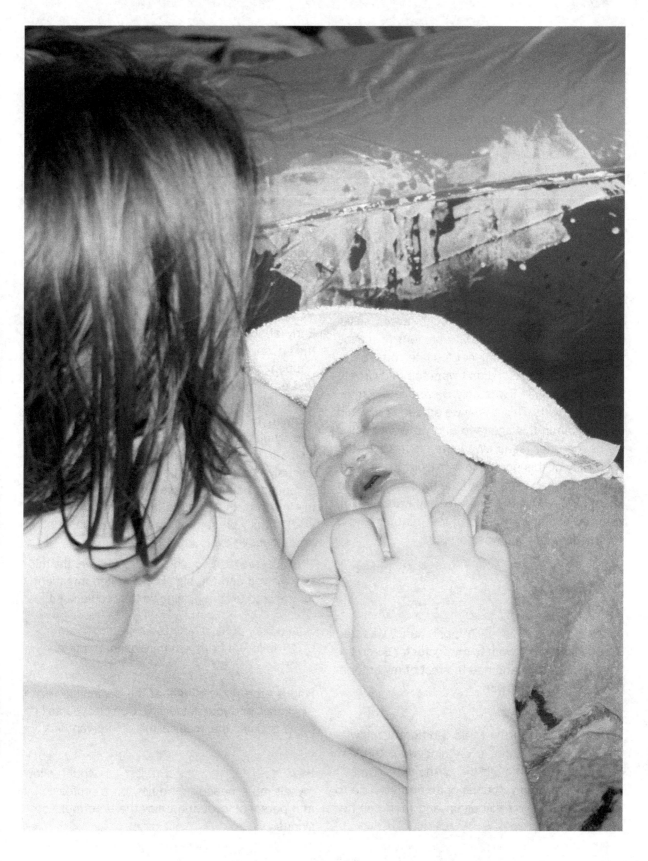

Self-Directed Pregnancy and Birth

Kathrin, 31
Job Title: Student

1st Child: Girl (6 y), birth in birth center
2nd Child: Girl (4.5 y), homebirth
3rd Child: Girl (3 y), homebirth
4th Child: Girl/boy (2.5 years ago), small freebirth at 11 weeks
5th Child: Boy (1.5 y), half planned freebirth

"Our little man was born with his whole family present, almost in the exact spot he now sleeps in every night."

When I hear the word 'freebirth', the following thoughts pop into my head: My favourite birth experience, love, family, oneness, calm, self determination.

When did you first have the idea to birth without a midwife? The birth was not planned 100% as freebirth, the first thought about possibly birthing without a midwife present or maybe taking the 'risk' of calling her too late came early, at around 12 weeks. I didn't want the midwife sitting around while I was only 3 cm dilated, making me nervous. This is why we agreed she would leave again in this scenario and we would call if we needed her (again).We were clear about the possibility of this ending in a freebirth and were ok with it. When I finally had the thought we could 'perhaps now call the midwife', my waters went, I started pushing and after a few minutes and 3 contractions our son was born.

Who did you tell of your plans? My husband, my midwife.

How did the pregnancy go and who did your antenatal care? The pregnancy was free of complications, I went to my doctor for 3 screening appointments and had the rest of my antenatal care with my midwife.

Why did you choose freebirth for yourself? For my previous births I had a different midwife and looking back, not everything went the way I wanted it to, although the births were lovely. I wanted to keep my options open and be able to call her, send her away again and then call her again if necessary.

How did you prepare for the birth? I read 'Ina May's Guide to Childbirth' by Ina May Gaskin and flicked through the 'Rockenschaub' (a German book on birth). I chatted with my midwife and husband and exchanged thoughts with other pregnant (freebirthing) women.

How did the birth go – any complications? Early labour dragged on a bit as I had an Au Pair in the house and it was hard to relax. Later, the birth happened calmly, without complications. For the first time I had no problems with an anterior lip of cervix. During the previous three births my cervix seemed to have been squeezed between baby and symphysis pubis, causing swelling and horrid pain. Good advice from my midwife and consciously changing position and staying 'upright' (kneeling) helped me avoid this problem during my fourth birth. Our little man was born with his whole family present, almost in the exact spot he now sleeps in every night.

The placenta came out quickly, just before the midwife arrived and the big sisters waited impatiently for the cord to stop pulsing so they could cut it.

How did you experience the postnatal period? In love, happy, calm, relaxed, nursing.

What would you tell other mothers-to-be? Find a good midwife right at the beginning. Listen to yourself and your gut feeling. Don't let yourself be pressured into the 'medical mill of interventions'.

What would you do differently during another pregnancy and birth? I would allow myself more peace and quiet, on a professional and personal level and enjoy the time more consciously.

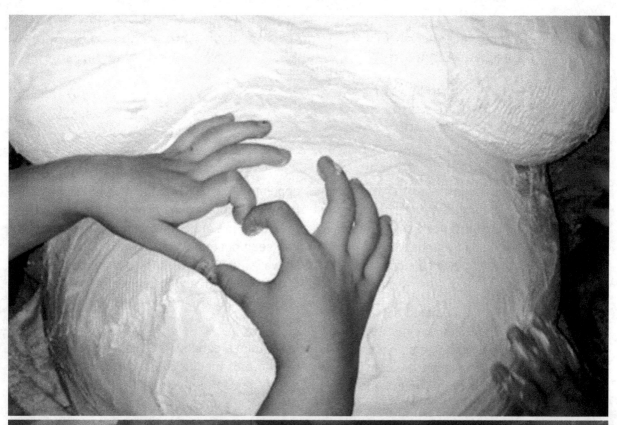

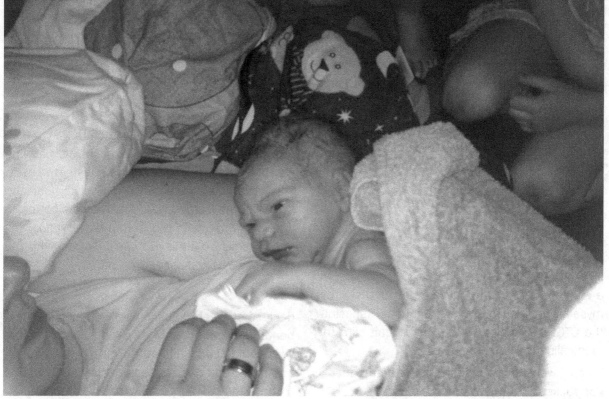

Tina, 32
Job Title: Almost finished at university
(European Ethnology)

1st Child: Girl (5 y), birth in birth center
2nd Child: Boy (3 y), freebirth
3rd Child: Boy (1 y), freebirth

"I found the processes I went through during pregnancy and birth very freeing."

When I hear the word 'freebirth', the following thoughts pop into my head: I like the term freebirth. I found the processes of pregnancy and birth very freeing. I have mostly freed myself from the feeling that I have to be monitored.

When did you first have the idea to birth without a midwife? I stumbled across a film of a freebirth from the US on the internet. Before that I thought it impossible that someone would remove themselves so far from the conventions around pregnancy and birth. Around the same time I fell pregnant for the second time. In the following months I first decided to explore freebirth in my dissertation for university, and then to also freebirth myself.

Who did you tell of your plans? Everyone who asked. Except for my doctor, but I stopped going to her at some point anyway.

How did the pregnancy go and who did your antenatal care? All three of my pregnancies went very well. In my first pregnancy I still went to my doctor for antenatal care a lot and to midwives once I had switched over to give birth in the birth center. After the birth I realised that the visits to my doctor always made me feel like I was ill despite feeling amazing and all test result being normal. In the second pregnancy I looked for a way to free myself from the expectations within myself. I declined lots of investigations, especially the CTG. Declining was the way I dealt with the medicalisation of antenatal care.

When I went to the doctor once, I automatically got sucked into the system of routine care, one appointment generated the next one. I cancelled the next appointment over the phone and felt relieved. I made contact with the midwife who I had seen postnatally after my first birth and got on well with. She was happy to come in the case of complications and to come after the birth otherwise. It was lovely to see her in the time after birth.

In the third pregnancy I realised the reservations I had towards medicalised antenatal care can't be transferred to all doctors. The doctor I saw this time (a different one) was very happy to accommodate my wishes, despite being surprised about how little care I wanted, which was only one ultrasound to determine the placental position.

It felt good not to see the investigations as compulsory but as an offer. My midwife was not working at that point. I found another one who was happy to support me but then had to withdraw her offer due to personal commitments, which was fine. After the birth I found a midwife who was happy to sign our papers to register the baby. This birth was very hard on my pelvic floor and I felt like my insides would fall out my bottom. I needed someone to reassure me everything was fine which is what this midwife did after giving me an abdominal massage.

Why did you choose freebirth for yourself? I decided on freebirth because I imagined it to be a beautiful experience. Most people I gave this answer to didn't find 'a beautiful birth' to be a strong argument, and not even something that could be in the same category as birth.

How did you prepare for the birth? My first birth in the birth centre was swift and gave me great confidence in myself. I simply knew I did birth well. I read a lot on the internet and read many books about complications and how to deal with them. From that I mostly learned that most risks are not actually a big deal.

How did the birth go – any complications? The first freebirth went well, though with 6 hours it was longer than my first birth as I was exhausted that evening. I could feel every contraction clearly, how the head moved through the birth canal and how the shoulders turned after the birth of the head.

My hands guided the fuzzy little head out, which felt amazing. I really didn't feel like giving birth during my second freebirth, and I told everyone loudly and clearly, which of course made no difference. Later when I wanted to push out the baby, progress stopped. I felt with my hand, and something was in the way. The baby had to move back up a little bit first and was then born without his hand by the side of his head. I'm not sure if you would call that a complication. I don't and was glad I was by myself, so no one could interfere.

How did you experience the postnatal period? The birth of a child to me is a process that lasts longer than the birth itself. Certainly in the first few days and weeks I had the feeling that the baby who was inside of me, was now on the outside of my body yet still a part of me. This process of 'severing the cord' still lasts to this day. The immediate post birth period is a very intense time for me as we adjust as a family in our new 'constellation'. My sister and house mates supported me in this time.

What would you tell other mothers-to-be? Giving birth is not as dangerous as people like you to believe.

What would you do differently during another pregnancy and birth? In another pregnancy I would have less negative attitude towards medical care in pregnancy and be positive about having the luxury to access investigations as and when I deem them necessary.

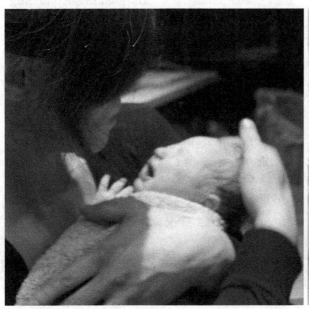
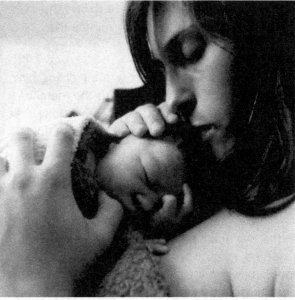

Sarah, 32
Job Title: Holistic healthcare practitioner

1st Child: Girl (10 y), homebirth
2nd Child: Girl (4 y), freebirth
3rd Child: Girl (2 y), freebirth
4th Child: Girl (3 weeks), freebirth

"Shortly after giving birth to my first daughter at home with the 'help' of a midwife I thought: 'Well, I could have done that by myself.'"

When I hear the word 'freebirth', the following thoughts pop into my head:

* A birth during which the birthing woman holds all responsibility (instead of looking for help while moving/looking away from herself)

* The woman knows what is best for her, has a connection to herself and her baby which leads her to the optimal birth process for herself and her baby.

* The woman decides herself what is good for her and her baby and is not disturbed by anyone – no comments, advice, interference, but also no thoughts or feelings from others (insecurities, fears, worries) that might influence her.

* Freebirth is for women who believe in themselves and who trust nature, life and themselves.

* To me personally, freebirth is connected to optimal birth – and a harmonious birth lays the foundation for a positive and happy human life.

When did you first have the idea to birth without a midwife? Shortly after giving birth to my first daughter at home with the 'help' of a midwife I thought: 'Well, I could have done that by myself.' And I think that the thought of doing it myself the next time was already formed then ...

I was 22 then and didn't really know that women did 'that'. But it somehow seemed normal to me.

Who did you tell of your plans? Pretty much at the beginning of the second pregnancy I knew I wanted to birth this baby in peace and quiet, meaning without any outside influence. I told my partner about my decision, who was happy with

it and also the singing circle that took place in my house at that time. There were no negative reactions.

I only found out a few months later that there is a name for births without outside help and was led to the book 'Unassisted Childbirth', which strengthened my convictions. I find it even more exciting that there will be a German book soon – thank you Sarah!

In the third and fourth pregnancy, everyone already knew of my plans. I have not received any resistance from anyone, but I do think carefully about who and how I tell my plans – I also don't tend to enter discussions as people who are not open to the idea don't change their minds anyway.

How did the pregnancy go and who did your antenatal care? During the second pregnancy I went to the doctor once for an ultrasound and saw the midwife a few times, but in a very 'hands off' way (no blood tests or vaginal examinations). I told her during our second appointment that I would like to do the birth myself, which was fine with her.

Seemingly, my decision led to debate in a midwifery forum though: Some midwives thought freebirth was a great idea, some thought it was 'off'. I signed a waiver saying I would take sole responsibility for the birth.

The pregnancies went well after the initial all day nausea.

In the third and fourth pregnancy I went for one ultrasound scan each and a midwife came once before the birth to lend us a birth pool. She also came two or three times in the days and weeks after the birth.

Why did you choose freebirth for yourself?
Simply said, it was a feeling, an impulse I was following! For me, it is the most normal thing I can imagine.

Some more specific reasons here:

* I don't like the fact that my midwife was the first person to touch my baby during the first birth and not me as her mother: she only caught my daughter and immediately put her on the floor so I could take her, but still, I found it irritating that a 'stranger' who would disappear from my life after the birth would be the first to touch my baby.

* She also got me out of the bath while I was pushing, and in retrospect it became clear I would have stayed in the bath had I been able to decide for myself: I wanted to avoid the danger of being 'directed' by someone else.

* I find birth to be very intimate and private, like sex. I don't want anyone around who tells me what to do or is 'only' watching. I am very clear about the influence the birth attendant's feelings can have on the process! Every outside influence has to be noticed, acknowledged or ignored. This takes time and strength, disturbing the birthing woman and bringing her 'out' of herself. Any disruption or disquiet disturbs the hormonal interplay which can cause complications or simply pain.

* Birth is the start of every (!) human life, and it doesn't have to be monitored.

* I'm more of a Do-It-Yourself-type and like to make my own decisions instead of following others!

How did you prepare for the birth? I read a lot in the first pregnancies. And because I am a homeopath myself and know a lot about the power of the subconscious mind, I have worked on and eliminated lots of negative thoughts and fears that came up by myself and the help of others.

In my third pregnancy I wrote down exactly what was important to me during birth and how it should be. This was really helpful to guide my thoughts into that direction during the birth, so I didn't think of things I didn't want but only the things I DID want (easy and joyous birth). '

How did the birth go – any complications?
All my births have gone well and happened without problems. To people looking in from the outside or in comparison to conventional hospital births mine seem to have been picture perfect.

However, for me personally, there was a difference in experiencing the process and in overcoming the 'pain'. With each birth I became more and more calm internally and I have experienced them more congruent with my own expectations of how birth should be (easy and joyous). I still think that each birth is a challenge to push your own limits – where the woman is asked to surrender, let go, trust and let things happen, simply and without resistance or control (which isn't for everyone).

The last two births were 'easy' – the only pushing contractions were the ones birthing the head and body. The first stages were not particularly painful for all births (comparable to slightly stronger period pains). I couldn't pinpoint transition with the last two births (apart from a brief thought). This is why I find it inappropriate to read how often contractions should be coming (!) to qualify for a certain phase of birth in some books: these thoughts can make birth much more complicated!

My second daughter was welcomed by my partner, who had lovingly and closely supported me during that birth, and put on my belly, and for the third and fourth birth it was important to me to consciously welcome my baby myself, which is how it happened!

During my second birth the 6 year old sister happened to be present which worked well. During the third birth I wanted to be without children – my third daughter was born during school hours and her 2 year old sister's daily 1 hour midday nap. With my fourth birth I thought she was going to be born during the night but she waited until the morning when all three girls could watch :-).

I like that my three daughters have experienced birth to be relaxed and easy!

And also something a bit more specific:

After the second birth I felt very stressed as the placenta didn't come immediately. This took away from the relaxed atmosphere we had (called the midwife, baby was crying) ...

So I decided for the next birth that the placenta would come when it's ready, be it after 1, 2 or 3 hours. It eventually came after 1.5 hours with a sudden and strong urge, and I was relaxed before and after, as much as I could be with afterpains anyway :-).

How did you experience the postnatal period? As a very special and thoughtful time, apart from some afterpains and mood swings :-)!

It can be an apprehensive time for the bigger children too, due to the many changes. So it can be helpful to have the partner present in the circle of family to be able to enjoy the new life, yourself as a woman and new mother and the special time in the partnership fully!

I have the wish that women would support each other again at this time (like in the olden days (?) or as social ritual) so that there can be even more relaxation and so that the time is seen and valued as something holy again!

What would you tell other mothers-to-be? Women, wake up! Be aware of your power and wisdom and take responsibility for yourself, your baby and your birth (otherwise someone else will)!

Widen your horizons in positive ways – birth can be so much more beautiful and easy than portrayed by many women, books and media!

Read good and lovingly written books, exchange information with other women who are aware and positive about birth. Explore your fears, perhaps even with outside help and be honest to yourself

(my tool of choice is EFT (Emotional Freedom Technique) which is great at eliminating blockages within yourself).

Learn to trust yourself, your impulses and your body and act like it! Stay true to yourself, even when people tell you differently during birth (or in life in general).

If you do want care in pregnancy, look for a woman who trusts your ability to give birth!

All the best for the readers and their children!

What would you do differently during another pregnancy and birth? Nothing!

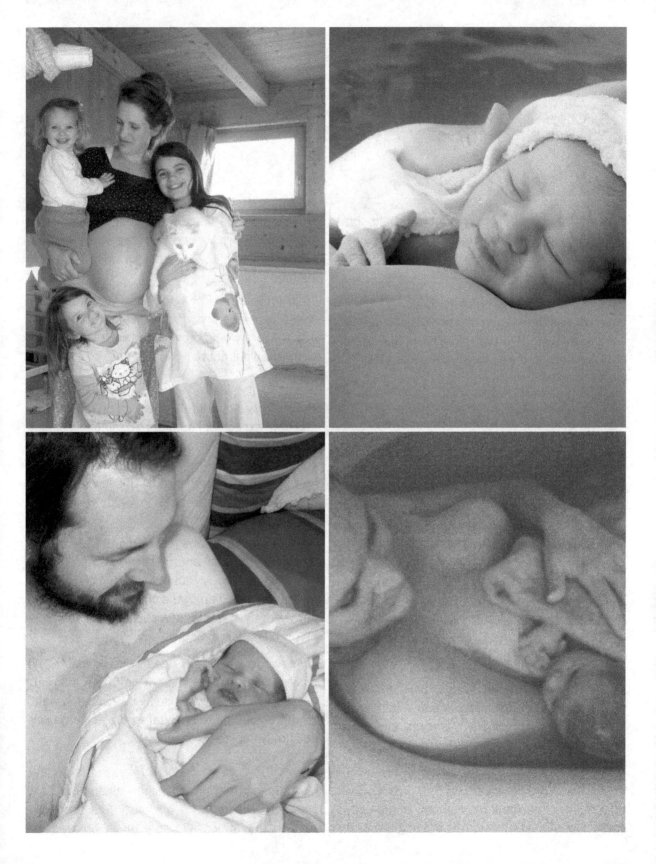

Self-Directed Pregnancy and Birth

Yvette, 32
Job Title: Family manager

1st Child: Girl (6 y), homebirth
2nd Child: Girl (4 y), homebirth
3rd Child: Boy (2 y), homebirth
4th Child: (6 mo), freebirth

"I relaxed with the knowledge that God would provide a pain free and uncomplicated birth for me."

When I hear the word 'freebirth', the following thoughts pop into my head: Calm, intimate time with God, my husband and baby, positive reaction from myself.

When did you first have the idea to birth without a midwife? Without me noticing initially, freebirth was the subject of a book I was reading. As I was thinking about pain free birth, this type of birth seemed to make sense. This was after the birth of my third child.

Who did you tell of your plans? I did not make a secret of my plans, except to the midwife.

How did the pregnancy go and who did your antenatal care? This pregnancy was better than the three previous ones. I had learned who God is since then and that He is good and carries our ills and pain (Jesaja 53:4), but that I have to accept this gift to me too.

So I started to grow in this consciousness and to act accordingly. During this I was able to experience a pregnancy without complaints, I didn't even need compression stockings – in my previous pregnancies I had always experienced severe oedema and pain. I only saw my midwife.

Why did you choose freebirth for yourself? I knew it would be easier for me to relax peacefully with God without any observers and other distractions. No professional would be able to irritate me.

How did you prepare for the birth? Apart from reading lots about the anatomy of the body I spent a lot of time with God, by reading the Bible, praying and singing for Him. Often during walks or cycle rides. In this time, while I was getting to know God better, I became so glad about Him that suddenly everything else (like a pain free birth) seemed unimportant.

I relaxed with the knowledge that God would provide a pain free and uncomplicated birth for me and that He would provide this in a subsequent birth, should it not happen this time.

How did the birth go – any complications? The birth was beautiful! Much, much more beautiful than expected. For about 20 minutes I experienced a sort of effort within my body, without feeling anything specific. Then I rested for an hour, first in bed, then in the bath. This is where I had my first (pain free) contraction, which was a pushing one right away.

Two more contractions followed and then my waters went suddenly and the baby came out. I felt this very consciously and caught the baby. I was rested and could enjoy the child with my husband immediately. It had a little suckle and then slept on my chest for an hour.

My newborns had never been this peaceful. The placenta came after another half hour following our prayer. The midwife had just arrived and wanted to transfer me to hospital as the placenta was still firmly in place.

How did you experience the postnatal period? Postnatally I was fit and well and our baby was very peaceful. He obviously had not experienced any stress. We very much enjoyed the time. Also, I hardly bled, and didn't immediately after birth either.

What would you tell other mothers-to-be? Matthew 6:33: "But seek first His kingdom and His righteousness, and all these things will be given to you as well." Here this means: Don't focus so much on the birth and what could go wrong, pain etc, but keep your eye on the living God who gives, blesses, loves, protects and spares us.

When we dedicate our life to God we don't have to expect or fear the curse of birthing pains – we can trust His proactive protection.

What would you do differently during another pregnancy and birth? I would grow more in my relationship with God and seek His kingdom, most importantly!

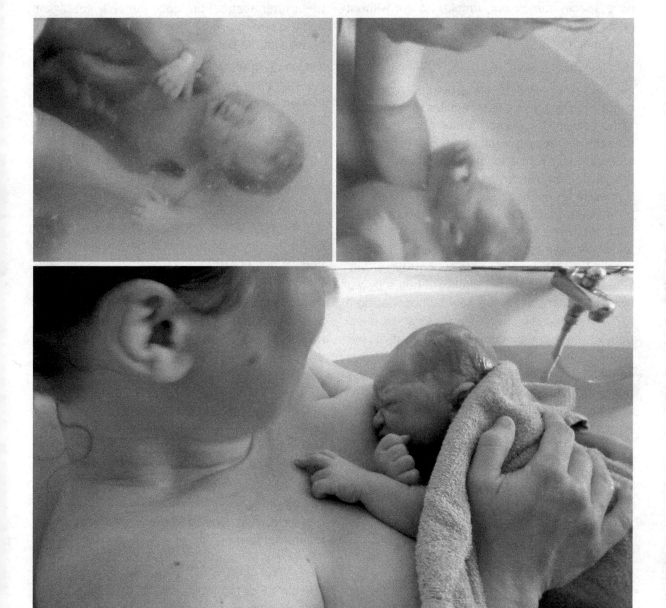

Rebekka, 33
Job Title: Engineer, last job: Manager Governance
in the Regional Government,
West Arnhem, Northern Territory, Australia

"The thought of freebirth intuitively felt right immediately."

1st Child: Boy (7 mo), freebirth

When I hear the word 'freebirth', the following thoughts pop into my head: I find the term 'freebirth' very appropriate. To be free, to have space, stretch out, unfold, let go, without other influence and prescriptions, pressure or time constraints.

When did you first have the idea to birth without a midwife? Long before I even became pregnant. I was very familiar with the idea of homebirth. I had read about freebirths. The thought of freebirth intuitively felt right immediately. Although I did discount the possibility for my first birth then. When I was pregnant I looked for a midwife for our homebirth. We had just moved from Queensland, where there are lots of homebirth midwives, to the Northern Territory. Here, midwives have very strict guidelines and for example, they are not allowed to support births outside of the bigger towns. We live 3 hours by car away from Darwin and the nearest hospital, so a midwife attended homebirth was out of the question. We considered all available alternatives (for example the birth centre) but the compromises connected to them proved too big. Freebirth was our next best option. Although it did take some time for me to accept that I was denied a midwife for my first birth.

Who did you tell of your plans? Only very few friends 'knew'. We live in a small village, my husband works in the local medical clinic and homebirths are most definitely not supported locally. But most people did figure it out, I think. At the latest, when I stayed in the village in the last few weeks instead of moving to Darwin as is usual.

How did the pregnancy go and who did your antenatal care? The pregnancy was one big miracle to me. Fascinating to see what our female bodies are capable of! In the first few months the thought of a baby growing inside me was rather abstract but once the belly got bigger and the baby started kicking – wonderful! I spent hours with the baby.

We hardly had any of the conventional testing, investigations and screening. This was a well informed and discussed decision. No ultrasound, no vaginal examinations, I didn't even weigh myself. I also did not see a doctor.

Why did you choose freebirth for yourself? Birth for me is an intimate family event and no medical emergency. This is why I feel the home is the most appropriate place to welcome a new family member into the world. Moreover birth is a finely tuned powerful process, on a physical, spiritual and emotional level.

I wanted to avoid any disturbance to this process and minimise the risk of complication that way. A homebirth was normal and a given for us. Even without a midwife.

How did you prepare for the birth? I have always been a sporty person, and I found it easy to maintain my fitness in pregnancy. Endurance training, weight training, Boot Camp, swimming, running, boxing, walking and lots and lots of yoga.

I also read as much as possible about pregnancy and birth, researched and exchanged information in internet forums.

How did the birth go – any complications? The birth was the most impressive, beautiful and exhausting event of my life.

Active birth started half an hour after my waters went. I was surprised at the immediate intensity of the contractions. I wanted to go for a walk and bake a cake! But proper labour had started and I had to concentrate fully on the contractions.

My partner and a friend who came for emotional support put up the birth pool, unfortunately it had a hole and we had a flood in the living room. I spent time in the bath and shower until everything had dried out.

After about 10 hours of intensive labour my cervix was fully dilated.

The second phase of birth was much more pleasant and beautiful to me. I wasn't aware of my surroundings anymore, I was away with the fairies. It took another 6 hours until our son was born. My partner was an amazing support and we really worked together as a team. He caught our baby when he was born.

I find it difficult to judge if there was complications, as my knowledge is solely theoretical. Nothing went obviously wrong. However I think that in the hospital, the length of the second stage would have been classed as a complication (and definitely would have led to intervention and possibly a caesarean section).

How did you experience the postnatal period? I was unbelievable happy that we were home and I could do what I wanted. I was off with the fairies and didn't want to come back to reality. It took us 2 weeks to leave the house. It was a very special time.

What would you tell other mothers-to-be? Don't hand over responsibility for your pregnancy, birth and baby to someone else. Be informed, ask, and consciously make decisions. It pays to go into pregnancy physically fit and healthy. And don't forget to enjoy the miracle.

What would you do differently during another pregnancy and birth? Nothing important. I would also like a birth with a midwife, but ONLY if she would respect ALL my wishes and I click with her 100% on a personal level. Otherwise I would have another freebirth. Perhaps with a midwife as back up.

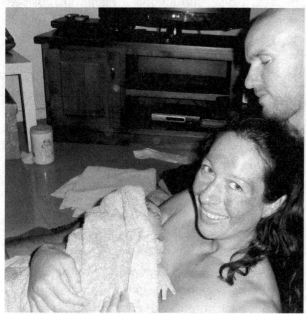
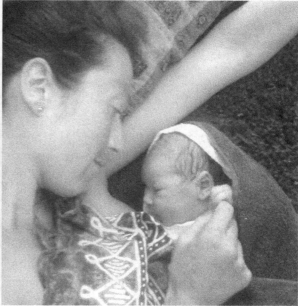

Romy, 33
Job title: Mother, musician, babywearing consultant, hypnobirthing teacher etc

"It was like the wave had swept me away, I was riding it and I knew, I was the wave rider."

1st Child: Boy (11 y), hospital birth
2nd Child: Boy (8 y), hospital birth
3rd Child: Girl (6 y), freebirth
4th Child: Boy (3 y), freebirth
5th Child: Girl (1 y), freebirth

When I hear the word 'freebirth', the following thoughts pop into my head: There comes a moment in every birth in which the woman realises that she is the only one who can birth this baby. Nevermind how many people are present, she is the only one who can make it a fulfilling birthing experience. The key for a dream birth is coming into your own power at that moment, taking full responsibility and directing the birth yourself. The essence of birth for me is found in freebirth and its potential to transform with its magical and spiritual magnitude, which enable the birthing woman to find her full female power and use it.

When did you first have the idea to birth without a midwife? During my second birth when I realised how people present and direction by others could influence my mood and the birth process.

Who did you tell of your plans? Only my husband.

How did the pregnancy go and who did your antenatal care? During my third pregnancy I looked for a midwife initially. The wish to birth alone only developed later in pregnancy. The midwife visited me at home once and felt for the baby's position. For my fourth and fifth births I let myself be guided by intuition and only got the midwife to confirm what I had already felt. My pregnancies were wonderful and intense at the same time, and I deeply engaged with the things important to me at the time.

Why did you choose freebirth for yourself? When I heard about freebirth for the first time I was fascinated. I imagined how I would surrender calmly and focussed on the gentle opening, together with my body and my baby. To surrender and to open is essential for birth. And many women, and I am one of them, do this best when they are alone or in the presence of loved and trusted ones.

A freebirth, under my own steam, without outside influence, seemed the logical and honest consequence.

How did you prepare for the birth? I prepared intensively on a daily basis, mentally, with affirmations, relaxation, breathing and other exercises. I also surrounded myself with positive people. I ate well and consciously treated myself to lots of peace and quiet and loving moments with my partner.

Furthermore, I kept fit with yoga and other exercise and listened to my body regularly. I had a deep bond with my baby.

How did the birth go – any complications? My three freebirths happened quickly, relaxed, beautifully and without issues. My third freebirth for instance: The mood in the room was mysterious. I lit candles, flowers everywhere. I relaxed, completely focussed and bonded with my baby. I was completely alone and yet I felt more supported and protected than ever. I breathed gently, focussed and guided my baby down the birth canal with each surge. With each surge she came a little lower and during each relaxing break I could feel her slip back up gently.

Though everything happened very quickly in the end I had plenty of time to relax. Everything became wider and wider. My daughter was on her birth journey, slowly but surely, until I felt the amniotic sac really close to my perineum. Opening became an even more intense sensation and then an incredibly intense power coursed through me, like an unbelievably powerful wave. It came from deep inside with such force, but pushed gently yet with amazing power.

The amniotic sac broke and I felt some hair. It was like the wave had swept me away, I was riding it and I knew, I was the wave rider and would not leave this wave. I breathed quietly but directed the breath through my body in the direction of the opening. I could see a flower opening her petals gently. I used my breath to guide her head gently over my perineum – as wide and open as possible – and then her head was there and she was making her first noises! I laughed loudly with joy

and happiness and with the next surge her body slithered out. I briefly took her in my arms and my heart and then my husband covered us both with a blanket and a hug. A moment in which time simply stopped. A magical and groundbreaking moment! Such an amazing birth heals old wounds and releases energy. Beyond generations and the universe.

How did you experience the postnatal period? I always found the postnatal period most beautiful at home. It was particularly valuable for the older children to be part of the early days. We were all able to experience this wonderful time together and it has shaped and nourished us.

What would you tell other mothers-to-be? Listen to your heart, your intuition, trust your body and take charge of your power. Every birth is a magical and deeply transformative event.

What would you do differently during another pregnancy and birth? Nothing.

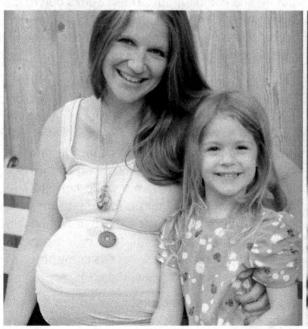
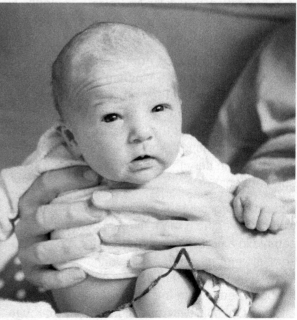

Stefanie, 33
Job title: Psychologist, Systemic Family Therapist

"I could already touch the bottom after the second pushing contraction."

1st Child: Girl (6 y), hospital birth (anthroposophical hospital)
2nd Child: Boy (3 y), half planned freebirth
3rd Child: Girl (6 mo), freebirth in breech presentation

When I hear the word 'freebirth', the following thoughts pop into my head: My own responsibility, trust, unhindered experience, connection.

When did you first have the idea to birth without a midwife? When I was pregnant for the first time. Then I thought about it out of fear of intrusive intervention. Now, because of my intuition and trust.

Who did you tell of your plans? No one for the second birth. For the third birth in breech presentation: my husband, my friend, my midwives (because of my husband) and my physical therapist.

How did the pregnancy go and who did your antenatal care? The second pregnancy was initially marred by the fear of developing preeclampsia again and that another haematoma could form in the birth canal and would have to be removed surgically. And also I would likely experience a retained placenta yet again and have a D&C after birth.

The doctor who looked after me recommended close monitoring and a planned caesarean section as 'that's what they are there for'. I then changed to an anthroposophical doctor who had operated on me after the last birth. She assumed that this pregnancy would be normal but still wanted me in her office for every other antenatal appointment.

The office procedure itself was unsettling to me: waiting, going from room to room, leaving a urine sample in a certain place, measuring blood pressure in another, then an examination and the 'expert hierarchy': the doctor apparently knew my body better than me. And then the torture of information: 'Oh, only one kidney!', 'not enough liquor', 'the baby is too low', 'the cervix is shortening'. All those were results I could ignore after researching them on the internet and listening to my body.

When I was supposed to turn up for appointments weekly because I was 'threatening premature labour due to my shortening cervix', I only went to my midwife for care. This was somewhat calmer until my blood pressure was borderline preeclamptic again towards the end of pregnancy (140/90). Two days after my due date our natural induction (prostaglandins in sperm support the opening of the cervix) was extremely successful. In my third pregnancy I finally trusted my intuition and declined antenatal care.

That turned out to be the best pregnancy of all of them! My husband wanted me to have a midwife, but I was hoping I would manage to have the baby before she could turn up. Three weeks before my due date I saw the midwife for the first time. She found the baby to be breech and said I should have 'a serious chat with the baby'.

This was a turning point for me. I had to support my intuition with knowledge. I researched night after night. I discovered that breech presentation only started to be classed as a 'malposition' a few decades earlier. Before that it was simply a rare but normal position for birth. I thought about the risks and how to minimise them. I could not find anything about breech freebirths in German speaking countries. Luckily there are women internationally who encourage women with their own experiences. The more I researched, the easier my husband found saying 'yes' to breech freebirth.

I also learned for the first time to feel for the baby's position myself. I wonder why women are taught how to check their breast for lumps but not how to determine their baby's position! As well as researching lots I also invited my baby to turn daily (Indian Bridge, rolling in the water, moxibustion, homeopathy) and said to him: 'It would be lovely if you could turn because I know how to birth a baby in that position. But I do think that any position you chose is the optimal position for you!'

Why did you choose freebirth for yourself? Because I trusted my inner voice and I didn't want to let the experts make me crazy again. In my first pregnancy, mild preeclampsia was diagnosed a week before my due date and the birth happened in the hospital due to that.

In my knowledge today I would still birth at home with such a condition as it can be classed as a normal process of starting to end the pregnancy as long as the blood flow through the cord is normal as intervention might lead to problems itself. In my third pregnancy the baby was the wrong way round. With such a malposition (breech) midwives are not allowed to attend due to insurance reasons. There is no way to get around that as the insurance companies and the government would go after them for damages in the case of anything going wrong ... she would have had to call an ambulance had I entered into a contract with her and declined transfer if she felt it appropriate.

Only very few hospitals let you 'try' to birth a breech baby vaginally. A waterbirth would be contraindicated as constant CTG monitoring would be impossible, getting a woman out of the pool may be problematic and doctors don't have easy 'access'. There would be an anaesthetist and doctor present during the birth, just in case. Birthing position would either be on my back or on all fours, if I didn't have an epidural anyway. Maneuvres to deliver the arms and head would be used even during an uncomplicated birth.

In German literature I could not find the English term 'Hand off the breech' while it is a common phrase in English midwifery literature. It means to not touch the emerging bottom during a breech birth. The birth attendant does not assist the

birth of the arms and legs. The head also does not get manipulated to turn with this method. The danger when touching the breech is that the baby startles, and moves one or both arms upwards which makes the birth of the head more complicated. So my wish for a natural, unhindered birth was only possible with a freebirth!

How did you prepare for the birth? With lots of information from books (Gaskin, Odent, Morgan) and the internet. Watched birth videos. Two videos made a particular impression on me, two mothers intuitively resuscitated their limp and blue babies at birth. This got me researching newborn resuscitation. I studied the statistics that made breech birth into a high risk situation. This showed studies have many faults but can still qualify as the basis for risk assessment in breech births.

Physically I prepared with deep breathing, relaxation exercises and perineal massage. Mentally I went inside myself and trusted my intuition. I also got a birthing pool. The water apparently minimises the chance of certain complications, such as cord prolapse especially during breech births. When the cord is visible but the head is not yet born, the baby may become distressed.

The time limits in which the head should be born vary greatly: from 2 seconds to 5 minutes! Due to the buoyancy of the water (from around 50cm depth), cord compression between pelvis and head is supposed to be less severe. Another danger is the potential stimulation of the breathing reflex when the baby's lower body is in contact with cold air. Amniotic fluid could enter the lungs. The warmth of the water is supposed to avoid this scenario and speed up the birth.

How did the birth go – any complications? Both freebirths: About an hour of contractions, about 10 minutes of pushing. No complications. The placenta came about an hour later in the squatting position I had moved into for birth. This is noteworthy as the placenta was expected to come out within 10 minutes after birth, while lying down, even in the anthroposophical hospital.

When this did not happen my uterus was manipulated, the cord pulled and oxytocics were administered. When it finally came out it was declared complete, which turned out to be wrong. A week later I had a D&C to get rid of remnants of the placenta. This was called 'retained placenta'.

With the second birth my contractions started around lunchtime. My husband finally called the midwives and I took off my trousers. That made pretty clear that we were not going anywhere. He was a bit worried and said: 'Slow down.' I said to him: 'I'd rather you said I was wide open!' To which he replied: 'You are as wide as the universe.' Then I had to push and my waters went, I kneeled down and the head was already visible. The head popped out with one last push. The little one immediately screamed. The cord was wrapped around him like a rucksack. We had to unwrap him to bring him to the breast.

The third birth started 6 days after my due date again around lunchtime. I walked up and down the corridor, breathing as per the Mongan Method through my surges and kept repeating the Gaskin mantra: 'I'm gonna get huge!' Then I got into the pool. At first I found that more unpleasant than walking around. So I told myself: This is the famous 'wanting to run away' feeling, things are starting to happen! I focussed on my mantra and breathing to keep contact with my primal brain. But then my neocortex took over and I felt to see if anything was there yet as I could feel the urge to push.

I could not feel anything. Was my cervix open at all? I only had a show about 15 minutes earlier. Then I remembered an e-book called 'Breechbirth'. A midwife was writing about women's intuition and that normally women with breech babies are told to resist the urge to push until the cervix is definitely fully open, but she had experienced (the only one as I recall) that it is better to follow the woman's intuition to avoid complications. Then I felt fear. Was I doing the right thing? And how would the baby fit? And what if this takes longer than the hour I had programmed into my self hypnosis? But then I remembered Odent and the necessity of fear. Fear

enables a release of adrenalin which in turn facilitates the fetus ejection reflex. So I judged this fear as something positive and could focus again on the process. I could already touch the bottom after the second pushing contraction. I turned from all fours into a squat (which is how the other births happened). The third push advanced the bottom considerably.

I had one hand on the side of the pool, the other on the baby's bottom. Despite the saying: 'Hands of the breech.' this is what I did intuitively. Oddly I could not feel any boy parts. Then the children started calling for me upstairs. I told my husband: 'Go. The baby will come by itself!' When he left the room, the fourth push birthed the body and head all in one go. I lifted the baby from the water and she cried immediately. The head was pink straight away, the body still a little blue.

My husband then came in, saw the baby, cheered and ran back upstairs to get the children. Both were really touched. It was a holy moment!

When I got out of the pool a few minutes later we called the midwife, we had agreed with her that she would write the birth notification to register the baby. Apart from the first examination of the newborn, we had no further check ups.

How did you experience the postnatal period? Very restful, no complaints apart from strong afterpains, but only very light lochia.

What would you tell other mothers-to-be? Go inside yourself, get in touch with your inner power. Trust your baby and your body. Inform yourself, face your fears and prepare mentally but also physically.

What would you do differently during another pregnancy and birth? I would be more confident following my female intuition and not tell anyone apart from my husband and physical therapist. Dealing with other people's fears is just too exhausting. I would want to be completely alone during birth.

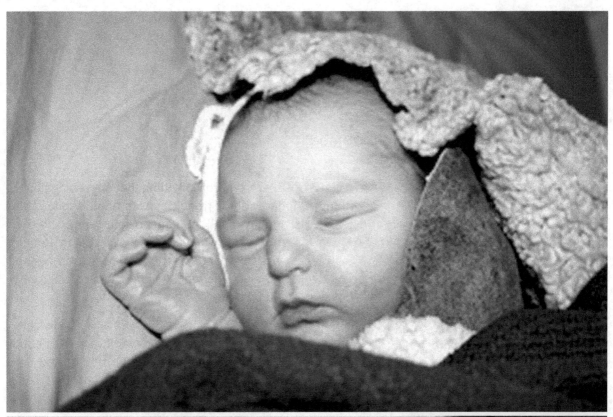

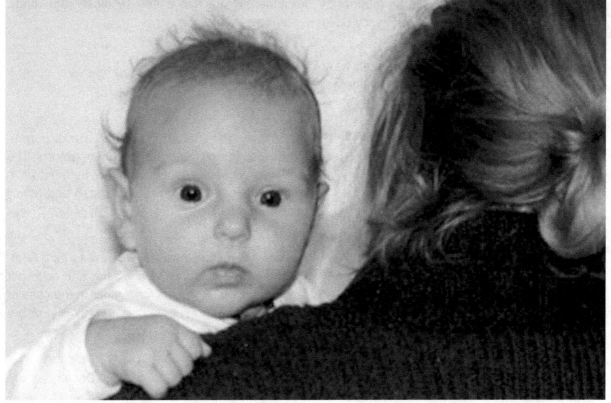

Self-Directed Pregnancy and Birth

Constanze, 35
Job title: Project manager

1st Child: Boy (9 y), hospital birth with early discharge
2nd Child: Girl (7 y), freebirth
3rd Child: Boy (5 y), freebirth
4th Child: Boy (2 y), freebirth
5th Child: on the way, freebirth planned

When I hear the word 'freebirth', the following thoughts pop into my head: Birthing naturally, freedom and responsibility, trust and instinct regarding your own body.

When did you first have the idea to birth without a midwife? During the second pregnancy. We planned a homebirth with a friend, a midwife who was only able to travel to Spain for the birth during a certain time period.

This is when I started (and didn't stop) to research what I needed to know in case I wanted to birth my baby alone (Freebirth stories, mostly from the US in those days, explanations in an internet forum by Dagmar Rehak and the Emergency Childbirth Catalogue).

It became clear that I could do it and really wanted to. And this is how it worked out: my friend was there but I did it myself.

Who did you tell of your plans? My husband, my family and my friend, the midwife.

How did the pregnancy go and who did your antenatal care? All my pregnancies went well, with my first I still went to the doctors for care. With the following three children and the one I am pregnant with now, I went for one ultrasound out of curiosity as I wanted to know if it was twins for the freebirths. Most of my support and strength came from my own research and the instinct within my own body.

Why did you choose freebirth for yourself? Why not? It is only one of many options of how to have a baby. Under normal, healthy circumstances there is hardly anything that speaks against it. Today, after 3 freebirths with another one in the planning I can't imagine any other way. The birth just happens while everyday day life carries on in a physically gentle and joyous way for mother and child. Husband and children are around, what could be better?

How did you prepare for the birth? To get in the mood for the birth I have always read about and watched videos on freebirth, and had little chats with the baby in my belly. I also found plenty of practical tips on the internet.

I generally practice a healthy lifestyle for body, spirit and soul.

How did the birth go – any complications? All my births happened quickly and without complications for mother and baby.

How did you experience the postnatal period? Postnatal period? I was whole, untraumatised, fit and well after all my freebirths. The baby practically slipped from my belly into the sling (while latched on to my breast) and family life continued.

What would you tell other mothers-to-be? Inform yourself extensively. Be aware that a woman actively gives birth to her baby, and does not get delivered by the doctor (except in the case of caesarean section or similar), her midwife or her husband.

What would you do differently during another pregnancy and birth? Document the process better.

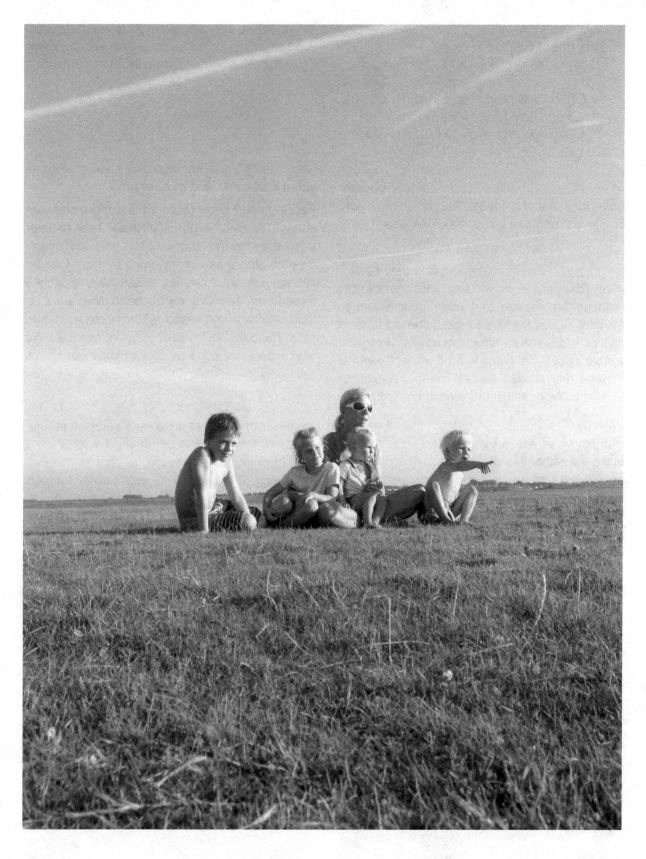

Jobina, 35
Job title: Life coach

"I sensually whispered 'Slowly, slowly!' to my baby and suddenly I was holding the tiny human bundle in my hands."

1st Child: Girl (7 y), birth in birth centre
2nd Child: Boy (2 y), freebirth
3rd Child: on the way, freebirth planned

When I hear the word 'freebirth', the following thoughts pop into my head: The most powerful moment of my life. Responsibility – power – love – truly being a woman/Goddess

When did you first have the idea to birth without a midwife? When my due date passed in my first pregnancy and the pressure from the birth centre midwife and other people around me grew stronger and stronger, I started to rebel internally against all time constraints. 'Everyone just go away – I'm going to do it myself!' was the thought that seeded my self-directed pregnancy and fabulous freebirth the second time round.

Who did you tell of your plans? Everyone who knew of the pregnancy. Lots of information was exchanged during chats when meeting people out and about. People assume they can ask everything regarding a pregnancy. However some found it difficult to deal with my definitive answers. There was some recommendations for doctors and midwives, and some critical questions. I used those questions for a reflective process. At first I sought answers in medicine and medical research but then I started to find all answers within myself. In my heart and my being.

How did the pregnancy go and who did your antenatal care? I did my own antenatal care. I took a lot of time for myself, as I was aware how much time I had saved by not going to any antenatal appointments.

Why did you chose freebirth for yourself? I felt safe. Even just the word 'Geburtshilfe' (which is the German word for obstetrics and translated literally, means 'help to birth') makes me feel like my ability to birth is in doubt. Birth does not need

help. I know my body best and know that I can guide it with my mind if necessary.

People I don't know (even if I find them pleasant enough) disturb me during birth as I have to enter a relationship with them. I have sensitive antennae for others and more empathy than I would like sometimes. I am not always able to protect myself from that. Only my husband deserves a relationship with me based on complete trust, surrender and the ability to open up at any level. We also experience this kind of opening in our sexual relationship.

How did you prepare for the birth? During the seventh month of pregnancy I started preparing daily, mentally and spiritually. I worked on a type of spiritual 'awareness' to change the programming of my first birth experience. I always focussed on a pain free birth, and kept this image in sight of my inner eye.

How did the birth go – any complications? I surrendered to all those finetuned processes within my body and accepted everything. I knew deep inside that my brain was my body's 'headquarters' and would look after every cell of my being and deliver the necessary biochemical cocktail (hormones) so that my feminine lower body could fully open to bring forth our child.

This is how I spent most of the first stage nearly alone and without anyone noticing. As soon as my husband appeared in my field of vision I started whining. I said I didn't want to do this anymore and could he please take over? When he said he hadn't even noticed things had started I told him to get a bucket. When I was promptly sick I realised in my head that I was in transition. The most exciting moment of this freebirth followed: LETTING GO.

I knew instinctively that I had to let go now, ignore my husband and put aside my personality/mind/ego. In that moment, when I closed my eyes and saw the words 'let go' written on the inside of my forehead, I felt as if I was turning into liquid. As if I was flowing into another state of consciousness. I lost all my sense of time and was floating in a fog of happiness. Then I felt the head passing over the perineum and almost enjoyed the feeling of fullness. I sensually whispered 'Slowly, slowly!' to my baby and suddenly I was holding the tiny human bundle in my hands.

My husband summed up the birth in one word: majestic.

How did you experience the postnatal period? I felt completely dignified and powerful as a woman and started everyday life overly eager. I had two or three days of the 'baby blues' where everything seemed too much and I felt alone. I had to learn to leave housework and to give my husband clear instructions. Physically, I experienced a fast recovery and a lovely breastfeeding relationship without problems.

What would you tell other mothers-to-be? Is there a more meaningful experience in a woman's life than the birth or a child? A self-directed birth enriches a woman's self confidence and self worth immeasurably. Lovely women, take back your wisdom and power of birth! It is in you, as much as you are female! Conquer your fears and don't constantly ask about risks and complications! Ask about what you can get out of it! Start to dream of your beautiful birth. You have to have a vision first, then it can become reality. You deserve it.

What would you do differently during another pregnancy and birth? As I am currently pregnant I'm preparing just as I have done previously. For the upcoming birth in summer I could imagine giving birth outside. Birthing as one with mother earth would be the only thing I might do differently.

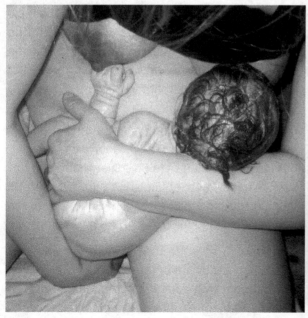 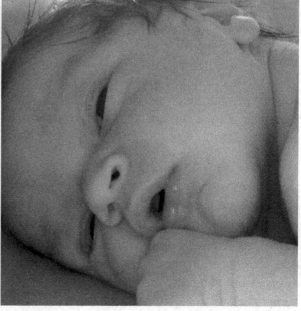

Nadine, 35
Job title: Author, coach for pregnancy, birth
    and time with the baby

1st Child: Girl (9 y), birth in birthing centre
2nd Child: Boy (7 y), freebirth
3rd Child: Boy (4 y), freebirth
4th Child: Girl (1 y), freebirth

When I hear the word 'freebirth', the following thoughts pop into my head: During all my freebirths I was physically completely alone, yet felt all the more supported and protected by beings from 'another world': birth angels, wise women and mother earth. These helped me to stay focussed on my centre, to keep the energies flowing through my body and gave me self confidence in the birthing process and my female power.

When did you first have the idea to birth without a midwife? After my first birth in the birth center which was lovely but very painful, I knew that it could be different. In absolute peace and quiet, complete relaxation and security, connected with very little pain and contractions, simply without any outside interference. It was clear to me I would most likely experience this by myself, which is how it turned out.

Who did you tell of your plans? Only my husband knew of the first freebirth. This birth was so easy and absolutely beautiful that with the following birth all our friends and family knew that I would only birth alone.

How did the pregnancy go and who did your antenatal care? In my second pregnancy I only had a couple of chats with the midwife but no examinations. In my third and fourth pregnancy I had no antenatal 'care'. I was healthy and rebalanced my body with homeopathy, oils, energy work and other method when I had slight complaints.

Why did you choose freebirth for yourself? I knew my body and myself very well and knew that I would relax and let go best by myself. This is the best prerequisite for birth.

How did you prepare for the birth? As I have described in my book 'Naturliche Wege zum Babygluck' I have prepared for freebirth with different methods. I was very creative, painted and made birth amulets.

As I could not find any German language information about freebirth and was a pioneer myself I read a lot in American yahoo groups and learned from other women's experiences. The American Laura Shanley has inspired me again and again with her book on freebirth.

How did the birth go – any complications? During all three freebirths and lotusbirths I experienced a deep calm and connection with the cosmos. They were easy, nearly pain free, and yet intense in their energy and primal power of birth – dream births that I will always carry in my heart.

Extract from my birth story: 'I could not see anything through the water in the gloomy candle light, but I felt for my baby. I felt a velvety head and tiny ears. What a miracle! I couldn't stop myself from laughing during the last two contractions and with the next contraction birthed our baby into my own hands, laughing.

I lifted him gently out of the water to my breast. In this moment I was one with creation and melted into my baby in a unity of pure happiness and unconditional love. I felt a breath of the universe and mother nature.

How did you experience the postnatal period? We had decided on lotus birth so the first few days were spent snuggling in bed. My husband looked after us lovingly after all my births and we were able to greet and enjoy the new family member together with the older siblings. I felt surrounded by and secure in a cocoon of love.

What would you tell other mothers-to-be? Birth is a formative and intense event for the baby as well as the mother. It is the first important imprint for the rest of life. Because of its importance I suggest to every woman to prepare well mentally and to create her optimal birth framework. Choose the place of birth and attendants carefully! I would recommend a homebirth with a loving midwife who carries the power and trust in birth and the birthing mother within herself to any healthy pregnant women.

What would you do differently during another pregnancy and birth? I'm almost certain that another baby would like to join our family. For me it is clear that it will be born at home and free again. Despite that I carry a longing for a birth in the ocean within me. I have read and written a lot about ocean birth with dolphins. Who knows, maybe I myself will be inspired by that.

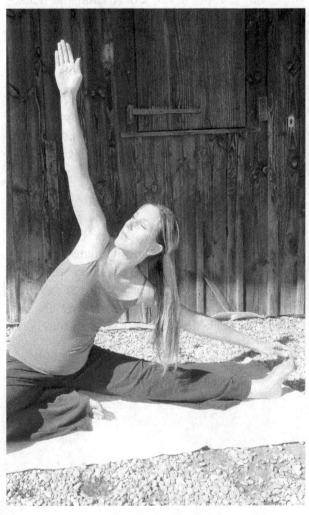
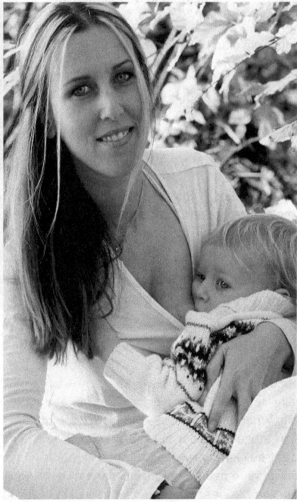

Uta, 35
Job title: Bookseller

1st Child: Girl (9 y), birth centre birth
2nd Child: Girl (7 y), homebirth
3rd Child: Girl (4 y), unplanned freebirth
4th Child: on the way, freebirth planned

"I visualised an opening lotus flower and breathed my third daughter into being pain free."

When I hear the word 'freebirth', the following thoughts pop into my head: Our freebirth was an unbelievably beautiful, strengthening experience which we will be eternally grateful for.

When did you first have the idea to birth without a midwife? The freebirth was not planned (it happened very fast and without complications), our midwife was simply too late.

Who did you tell of your plans? No one because we didn't have any plans.

How did the pregnancy go and who did your antenatal care? We switched between doctor and midwife for our antenatal care. In the last trimester we attended a hypnobirthing course.

Why did you choose freebirth for yourself? We didn't have a choice – but despite that it was one of the best and most empowering experiences of my life.

How did you prepare for the birth? With all the wonderful hypnobirthing practice and particularly the daily rainbow relaxation.

How did the birth go – any complications? I woke up around 4am with regular surges. At 4.45 I woke my husband and after the 'bath test' the contractions were so powerful that I was struggling to cope as I was using the 'wrong' breathing. When I finally realised that this was not the first stage of labour but the second, everything went quickly. I visualised the opening of a lotus flower (and nearly sent my husband away to find tea compresses for my perineum – luckily I called

him back straight away!) and breathed my third daughter into being pain free. She was born in a splash of amniotic fluid directly into the arms of my love, for whom this freebirth was a huge gift as well.

How did you experience the postnatal period? It was a dreamily quiet time with lots of snuggles, completely removed from everyday life: my lovely parents in law looked after the household and older siblings for a month, my husband took holidays and we had loads of time to get to know our youngest addition.

What would you tell other mothers-to-be? Believe in your power and wisdom: Your body knows how to birth a baby gently, safely and without pain – trust Him and the heavenly powers and surrender to the primal forces during birth. Have trust! In yourself and your baby.

What would you do differently during another pregnancy and birth? My preparations for birth were perfect. For the next birth I dream of the attendance of my favorite midwife and my friend (who is a student midwife): they will be allowed to sit in the garden and drink tea, because really, I would like another freebirth with my love – but I would like the feeling of security they could give me just by being there.

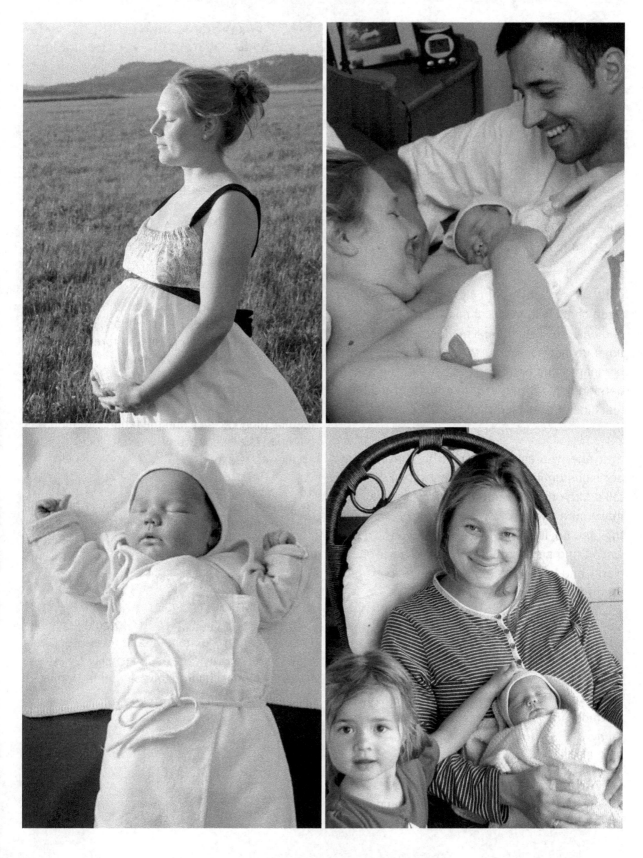

Self-Directed Pregnancy and Birth

Beatrice, 36
Job title: Adult education, mother

1st Child: Girl (5 y), freebirth
2nd Child: Boy (2 y), freebirth

"I was ready to take responsibility for my family from the very beginning."

When I hear the word 'freebirth', the following thoughts pop into my head: Peace, responsibility, family, independence, awareness, quiet, life changing experience, fulfillment, universal support, friends, unity

When did you first have the idea to birth without a midwife? In my first pregnancy I had three chats with my local midwife. After the second one I realised that all the tests and examinations do not contribute to a healthy and joyous pregnancy and birth. I only felt stress and misunderstanding. I didn't want to be part of the 'birth machine'. So I did it myself.

Who did you tell of your plans? The first time everyone who asked. I wanted to challenge my decisions until the end and strengthen them. In talks with others I wanted to discover myself and make sure I was not on some sort of weird ego trip. And no, it definitely wasn't an ego trip. I convinced and surprised myself with assertiveness, clarity and love. I was ready to take responsibility for my family from the very beginning.

How did the pregnancy go and who did your antenatal care? Both pregnancies went well. No one found anything abnormal and I felt free and happy. I read a few books, watched birth DVDs and often retreated into myself. Silence is my most trusted and constant companion until today.

Why did you choose freebirth for yourself? I felt it was too risky to have a midwife present. In the end she might rescue herself and not me. This is fact, looking at the current litigious climate.

How did you prepare for the birth? I was introspective. Painted intuitive pictures about the baby's position, process of birth, inner attitude and possible hindrances. Dreams provided me with information such as the baby's sex, readiness and expectations.

How did the birth go – any complications? Both births were quick and to the point. Every moment burned itself into my heart, joyously and clearly. Both times my perineum tore 6-8cm and healed without problems by itself.

How did you experience the postnatal period? The first time round it was stressful, breastfeeding didn't go well and the family situation was difficult. The second time we had local support and it was relaxed.

What would you tell other mothers-to-be? Be still and calm. Check everything you hear, diagnoses and rumours and follow your inner path. Birth is what we are made for. Birth means becoming a woman and discovering the roaring lioness within yourself. Enjoy it!

What would you do differently during another pregnancy and birth? I would keep everything open in the moment and revise decisions again if necessary. The responsibility I will hold myself – for my children, myself and my family.

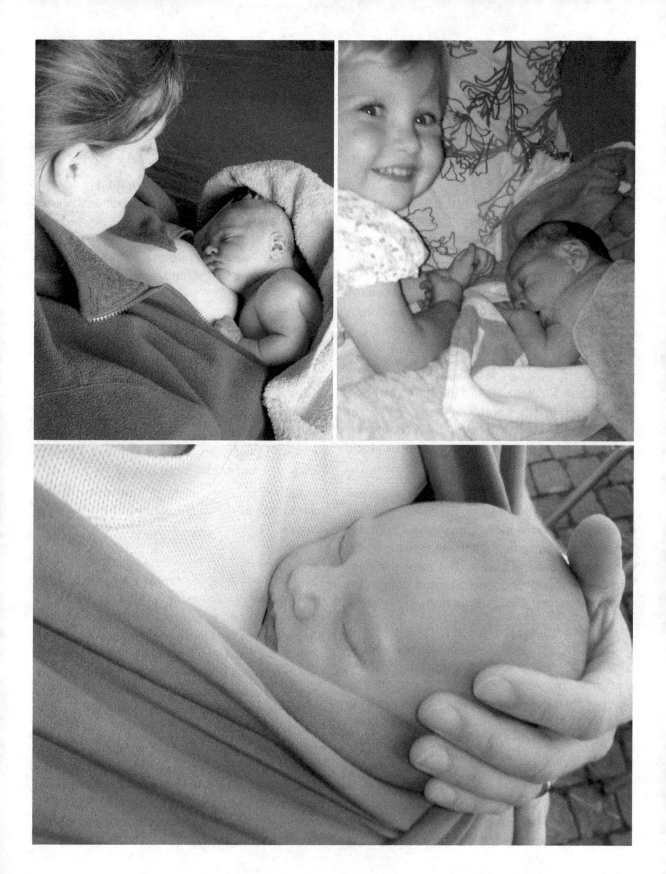

Caroline, 37
Job title: Musician, author

"My husband stood in the bathroom about a minute after the birth, sleepy and amazed."

1st Child: Girl (8 y), hospital birth, caesarean section
2nd Child: Girl (6 y), homebirth
3rd Child: Girl (10 mo), freebirth

When I hear the word 'freebirth', the following thoughts pop into my head: Wonderful! I already thought with my first child this would be the best option for me. Unfortunately, I wasn't quite intuitive enough then and let others influence me with their talk. I paid for my heedlessness with an unwanted caesarean section which was difficult to cope with and estranged me from my own body.

When did you first have the idea to birth without a midwife? A while ago when I read about Sarah's forest birth in 'Luxus Privatgeburt'. I had already had my homebirth then and thought to myself: Completely without midwife, that would be the crowning glory. If perhaps not on a picnic rug in the woods.

Who did you tell of your plans? First just myself. Then the baby. Then my husband. Then my daughters. I wanted everyone to know that I was hoping they'd sleep through the birth after all. Except for the baby of course. But even the baby was only active for about an hour and then saved her strength for the exhausting part.

How did the pregnancy go and who did your antenatal care? The pregnancy went by without complications. I exercised a lot (yoga) and on the day before the birth I swam a whole kilometre. I did my own antenatal care, only spoke to my trusted husband about some specific issues and phoned/emailed my homebirth midwife. I met her once. I did not have any checks.

Why did you choose freebirth for yourself? I always felt this was a fantastic option for me. As a musician I am used to focussing on myself and also know how easy it is to be distracted. Es-pecially during the birth I didn't want any distractions, and getting the midwife to attend (she lives very far away) with two children etc etc seemed too much effort with the third baby. This would have unsettled me before the birth already as I didn't know when the baby would decide to be born.

How did you prepare for the birth? By growing a thick skin against the stupid comments about pregnancy from outsiders. Especially the question: 'When will the baby come?' got on my nerves and I finally used the answer: 'When it's done'. I was very careful with my nutrition and mostly eliminated sweets, flour, bread, pasta, rice etc – and I kept very active, like I said. I gained 6.5kg and my baby weighed 3kg.

My baby is a yoga baby even now, it seems she internalised all the yoga movement from the pregnancy.

How did the birth go – any complications? The birth was free of complications and quick, from my waters releasing around 1.30am I laboured for 3 hours, only one of which was actually hard work. Just like during the second birth, I went to the toilet and firstly emptied my amniotic sac, then my bladder and finally my bowels (without an enema, my body takes care of it itself) and then prepared for productive contractions which promptly started.

Most of the birthing time I spent in our little bathroom, and circled my baby down with the appropriate (circular) hip movement and helped her into the right position. I also noted down my progress. For the last note I only managed to write down the time.

Then things really started to progress and I did everything right, without outside help. I just knew what to do and I cheered my baby on loudly during the last few big surges: 'Come on, help me, two more contractions and you are here!' As per my wish, my family did not disturb me at all.

My husband stood in the bathroom about a minute after the birth, sleepy and amazed. He thought the noise he could hear was from the flat above us. Initially I could not answer his question if it was a boy. I was still counting fingers and toes and checking if the palate and back were intact and closed. Then our two dogs came into the bathroom, and after that – with a flashlight – the two big sisters. When they first got sight of the baby I heard a 'ewwwwww' which was in response to the vernix.

After the birth of the placenta (I pushed and at the same time gently pulled it out about 15 minutes after the birth) I chewed through the umbilical cord. Later I noticed an excessive loss of fluid with lots of mucousy lumps and mostly blood. I was unsure of what this might be and called my midwife. She said to check the placenta very carefully and to send her a picture of it.

On the picture it was obvious the placenta was complete. But we could see the place where a second placenta had been attached, and when I fished the pads out of the bin I could see a partly reabsorbed, necrotic second twin. My suspicions from early pregnancy that I would have two babies were confirmed. This also explained the great sadness I felt around the 20th week of pregnancy.

How did you experience the postnatal period? Ecstatic, proud, somewhat hyper, but also extremely tired with a need to sleep. Luckily my husband often sorted the bigger girls in the morning so I could stay in bed with the baby. I quickly started exercising again and occasionally overdid it. What's good about that is: when my batteries are empty my body forces me to rest anyway.

What would you tell other mothers-to-be? Trust your feelings and ask 1000 questions when it comes to the birth of your baby. Good births are not easy to find, only the best is good enough for you! You don't give birth often. It is worth it to prepare carefully and only take people who you trust 100% into your confidence.

What would you do differently during another pregnancy and birth? Compared to the last birth? Nothing! Everything was perfect.

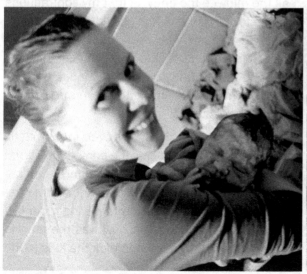
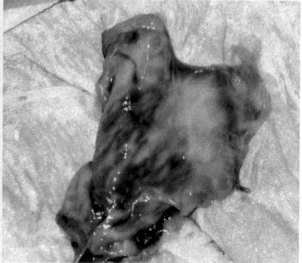

Self-Directed Pregnancy and Birth

Franziska, 37
Job title: Care worker

1st Child: Girl (6 y), hospital birth with early discharge
2nd Child: Girl (4 y), birth in birth centre
3rd Child: Boy (14 mo), unplanned freebirth/planned homebirth

When I hear the word 'freebirth', the following thoughts pop into my head: ... the amazed faces when we tell people about our birth experience and my husband reports he did everything himself!

When did you first have the idea to birth without a midwife? I never had the idea. It just happened that way without me ever thinking about it.

Who did you tell of your plans? All the people close to us (family, friends, neighbours) knew we were planning a homebirth.

How did the pregnancy go and who did your antenatal care? My pregnancy was free of complications. However from the fifth month I suffered lots of pain from symphysis pubis dysfunction which did dampen my joy in this pregnancy somewhat. My antenatal care was done by the same midwife I had during my second pregnancy, birth and postnatal care. So U. was a trusted person for the whole family. All my antenatal appointments were done in our home with our two girls present. I could chat about all my little worries with U. and felt very well looked after.

Why did you choose freebirth for yourself? I planned a homebirth with my midwife really. The situation was as follows: The birth centre I used to give birth to my second daughter and where I really felt at home had closed down. A birth in the hospital was unthinkable for me. So I had no other choice and had to convince my husband that I wanted to give birth at home. That was hard work, but I managed it. But then everything happened differently to how we imagined it anyway.

How did you prepare for the birth? In the summer holidays I read 'Ina May's Guide to Childbirth' by Ina May Gaskin. This encouraged me to trust in myself and my baby. I practiced pelvic floor exercises and pregnancy yoga throughout the whole pregnancy.

Three weeks before the birth we put up the birth pool in the bedroom and put together everything we might need. I think when a couple plans a homebirth, the preparations are automatically much more intense than with a hospital birth. I had to decide consciously who I wanted to share the intimate and formative moment of birth with. And I also imagined exactly which room I wanted to birth in and what the atmosphere should be. Every night when I went to bed I imagined how I soon would be in the pool, giving birth to my baby.

How did the birth go – any complications? The birth started during the night. I didn't want to call the midwife too early so that my contractions would stop again, so I just stayed in my bed and breathed joyously with every contraction. I had enjoyed experiencing the first surges together with my baby in my second pregnancy as well. When the alarm woke my husband in the morning I told him my secret.

Now the peace and quiet was over. In the hectic excitement he started filling the pool. Our children woke up, filling the house with life. In the meantime my waters went. Contractions now came frequently and strongly. I paced the living room like a tiger in a cage. I thought now was the time to call the midwife. My husband took the kids to the neighbours' house.

As soon as they left the house I went upstairs – and felt I needed to push. The pool was only half full. 'The baby is coming!' I said to my husband. He panicked and called U. again. She was on her way but stuck in morning traffic and only moving slowly. 'Just give birth', I heard her say over the phone. I was still standing, leaning over the side of the pool. Things were serious. With the next contraction I could feel the head. 'Everything is all right.'

I tried to calm my husband. And then the head was out. For a short moment I thought: 'I hope it's alive!' It seemed to take an eternity until the next contraction that pushed our son into the world! He was welcomed by his father's hands and then I was able to say hello. Finally I sat down on the bed, the naked little bundle in my arms. This is when U. entered the room. Now I could relax and she took care of everything else. She put a blanket over us, cut the cord and helped with the placenta. Soon after our two girls greeted their brother.

How did you experience the postnatal period? In the first few hours I was just so happy that our midwife made sure me and the baby were skin to skin in our little nest. She insisted I create little 'islands' so I could be alone with the baby. My husband and mother mainly looked after the bigger children in the first two weeks. The 'Spitex' (hospital provided home help in Switzerland) sorted the household.

What would you tell other mothers-to-be? The less technology is used for pregnancy and birth, the more confidence the woman will have in herself and her body. A natural birth with trusted people around her is a wonderful experience that can provide a woman with long lasting strength and energy. It does matter how we are born. The pregnancy influences birth which in turn influences the initiation of breastfeeding. All this is the basis for a positive mother-child relationship.

What would you do differently during another pregnancy and birth? I would make sure there was less pressure and stress during pregnancy so I could enjoy the time more. The birth was just beautiful.

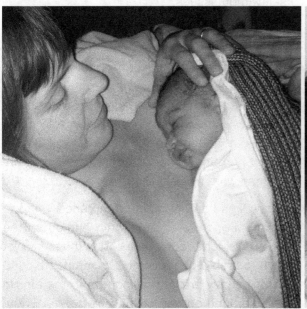
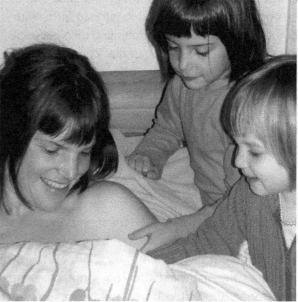

Self-Directed Pregnancy and Birth

Yvonne, 38
Job title: Commercial employee

1st Child: Boy (11 y), homebirth
2nd Child: Girl (8 y), freebirth
3rd Child: Boy (7 y), freebirth

"The memories of our first birth, when I nearly bled out because our midwife pulled out the placenta too soon, overcame me."

When I hear the word 'freebirth', the following thoughts pop into my head: Familiarity, being at home, self-directed, intimacy, freedom, responsibility

When did you first have the idea to birth without a midwife? When I was pregnant with my second and midwives wanted to restrict my freedom with interventions.

Who did you tell of your plans? My husband.

How did the pregnancy go and who did your antenatal care? All my pregnancies went well, apart from common complaints like oedema, heartburn and backache. In my first pregnancy I went to the doctor mostly, in the second pregnancy I went to the midwife a few times and in the third I hardly saw either of them.

Why did you choose freebirth for yourself? I chose this type of birth for myself because I wanted complete freedom when it came to birth, without limitations or interventions and also because my midwife pulled the placenta from my uterus far too quickly (12 minutes after birth) during my first birth, resulting in a heavy bleed.

How did you prepare for the birth? I read many homebirth stories that made me trust in me and my body, but also hospital birth stories that put me off.

How did the birth go – any complications? First freebirth: Now and then the memories of our first birth, when I nearly bled out because our midwife pulled out the placenta too soon, overcame me. The same midwife did my antenatal care and threatened she would have to put a venous ac-

cess in and have a second midwife present. No! I definitely did not want that and decided to birth alone.

Around 5am, 8 days past my due date, the first surge. I quickly sorted out pets, and my husband filled the birth pool.

The water made the surges much easier to bear. With two overwhelming pushing contractions that flowed into one another my waters went and the baby shot out of me. I gently pulled the little one out of the water, she was beautiful. Immediately she turned blue and coughed. A frightening moment that chilled me to the core.

Instinctively I grabbed the cord. It was still pulsing and I felt calmed as she was still getting oxygen. My daughter stayed attached to the cord for over an hour, and the cord kept pulsing until we cut it. This time the placenta had enough time to detach itself without issues.

With the next birth I asked my husband again to fill the pool but the surges continued only coming every 20 minutes. I lost my patience. Shortly before 7 o'clock I got into the warm water and it was as if a switch had been thrown. Surges every 2 minutes. Around half seven the urge to push. Our son shot out of me like an arrow, just like his sister. Short and powerful. At first I could not understand what I was seeing.

My son was born in intact membranes. I had to tear them open to be able to lift him out of the water. The membranes were soft to the touch, yet tough to break – I needed to use proper force to do so. I gently brought my son up to the air. He looked around and at me with alert eyes. Everything was so peaceful. After 20 minutes I passed him to my husband after he had cut the cord.

I birthed the placenta in the water without any problems, got out of the pool and snuggled down with my third born. Shortly after his two siblings woke up and greeted their brother with amazement.

How did you experience the postnatal period? In my first postnatal period I was exhausted due to blood loss and got terrible mastitis, but recovered quickly. Apart from that I was ok, but felt a little unsure of myself. I fell into a routine more each day. I experienced the other two postnatal periods as positive.

What would you tell other mothers-to-be? Take responsibility for yourself and determine your own path through pregnancy and birth. Have trust in your body and your ability to birth a baby.

What would you do differently during another pregnancy and birth? I would not have any antenatal care and birth by myself again – the more natural the better!

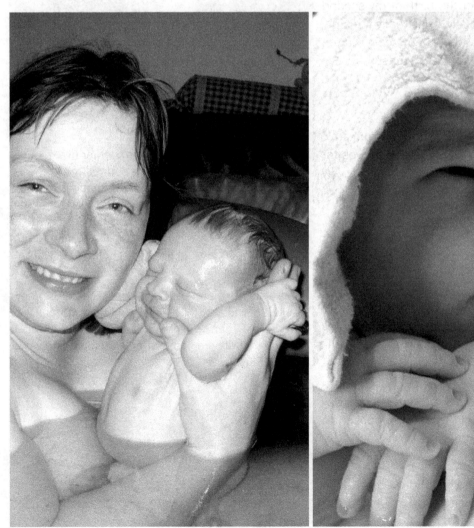
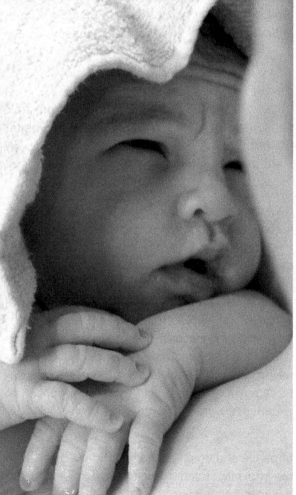

Self-Directed Pregnancy and Birth

Angela, 39
Job title: Architect

"My third child was not supposed to experience what the first two had to."

1st Child: Boy (9 y), hospital birth, caesarean section
2nd Child: Boy (7 y), hospital birth, ventouse birth
3rd Child: Girl (4 y), half planned freebirth

When I hear the word 'freebirth', the following thoughts pop into my head: To have peace and be left alone. Take responsibility, go into birth consciously. Being present, being in control of my body, to be able to let go, without obstacles.

When did you first have the idea to birth without a midwife? After the birth of my second son but only subconsciously. I was really thinking: 'Enough. I'm not going to let them cut me open again in the hospital without good reason.'

Who did you tell of your plans? Nobody.

How did the pregnancy go and who did your antenatal care? I had care from 'my' midwives and friends. I did pay the midwives for the birth too but really, I knew I wouldn't actually need them.

Why did you choose freebirth for yourself? It was never a conscious decision or one I ever verbalised, but when the birth started I didn't feel I needed anyone. I just wanted to be alone. Because I wanted to remain whole and wished for a normal birth, finally. And mostly because I knew that the caesarean section with the first and the ventouse and episiotomy with the second baby were not really necessary. I also didn't want to be separated from my baby without good reason (I saw my son for the first time on the second day after birth). My third child was not supposed to experience what the first two had to.

How did you prepare for the birth? With lots of peace and quiet, I literally withdrew from life in the end. I lied happily when necessary and took a daily lunchtime nap!

How did the birth go? Any complications? No problems. I woke up in the middle of the night and my contractions started gently and slowly. After about an hour I woke my husband to tell him that perhaps he should not go the airport ... and went back into the kitchen. A kitchen birth, not very romantic, but it was simply the best place. I found some baked treats and was happy.

I was doing well, the contractions were not painful. Until I noticed I was unable to read the time ... and opened a cookbook. I was on my journey, the ravioli jumped out at me, the mussels opened up, everything seemed to be moving around and reminded me of vaginas, it was somewhat intoxicating. My husband then came into the kitchen and we wondered for a while if this was proper labour or not.

He called the midwife but after another five minutes I suddenly wanted to go to the bathroom and there I could only hold on to the door and shout for my husband so he could take off my trousers. And then the baby was already there. He had his hands in the right place and then he was just sitting there, in our bathroom between Playmobile ship and kid's socks, with our baby in his hands. Wonderful.

The placenta came out right after. The big brothers woke up and stood behind the bathroom door with wide eyes! Then we got into our big bed and waited for the midwife. The days after were the best, just at home. Plus it was Christmas!

How did you experience the postnatal period? It was fantastic.

What would you tell other mothers-to-be? Ask questions about everything. Anything at all!

What would you do differently during another pregnancy and birth? Even more peace and quiet.

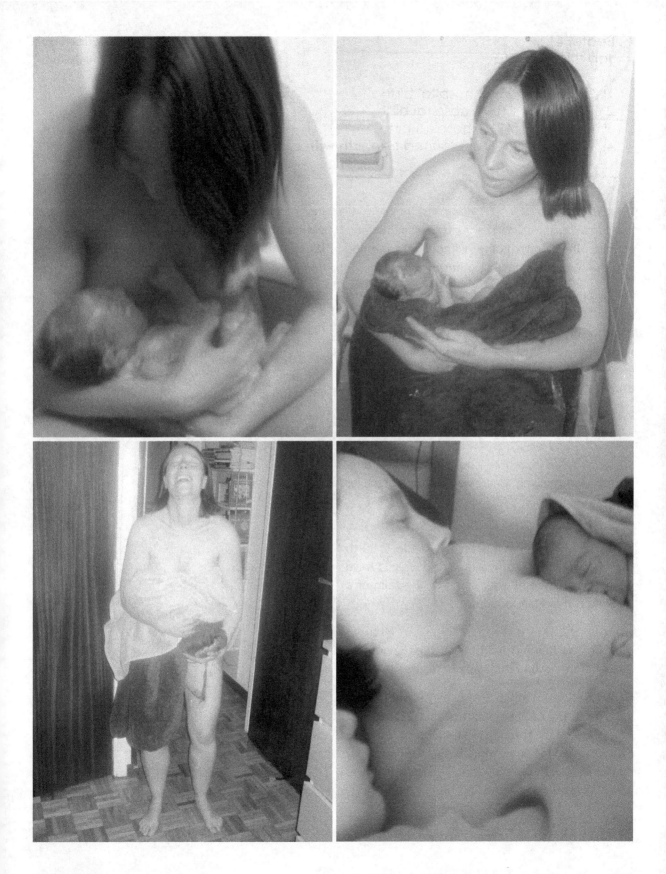

Beate, 41
Job title: Midwife

**"There were no complications
and for the first time, no tears."**

1st Child: Boy (25 y), hospital birth
2nd Child: Boy (21 y), hospital birth
3rd Child: Boy (12 y), hospital birth
4th Child: Girl (4 y), unplanned freebirth with planned home birth

When I hear the word 'freebirth', the following thoughts pop into my head: self-directed birth in my own home, without interference into the natural process by others.

When did you first have the idea to birth without a midwife? I would have liked a homebirth for my third birth. With my fourth child I finally planned to just call a colleague for the birth if needed. I intended for her to be there – preferably in another room.

Who did you tell of your plans? My husband.

How did the pregnancy go and who did your antenatal care? Lovely pregnancy, supported by a midwife, I only went to my doctor for an ultrasound.

Why did you choose freebirth for yourself? Because I know that women are made to birth their babies all by themselves. It is lovely to have a trusted midwife by your side – if the help of a midwife is indeed needed.

How did you prepare for the birth? I am a midwife and had birthed three babies spontaneously before my daughter was born.

How did the birth go – any complications? Very! Fast. My baby was born within 28 minutes from the first contraction. The speed of the birth overwhelmed me somewhat, but all went well! My husband caught our daughter :-) There were no complications and for the first time, no tears.

How did you experience the postnatal period? It was very relaxed and wonderful. It is just so lovely and relaxing at home. I had a lot of peace and quiet despite the other kids. My husband managed to keep visitors away from me.

What would you tell other mothers-to-be? If possible, have your baby somewhere other than a hospital. If this is not possible, try to get an early discharge.

What would you do differently during another pregnancy and birth? I would do everything the same :-)!!

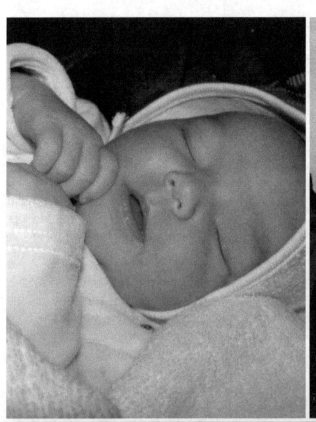

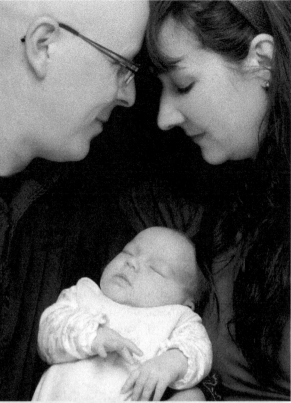

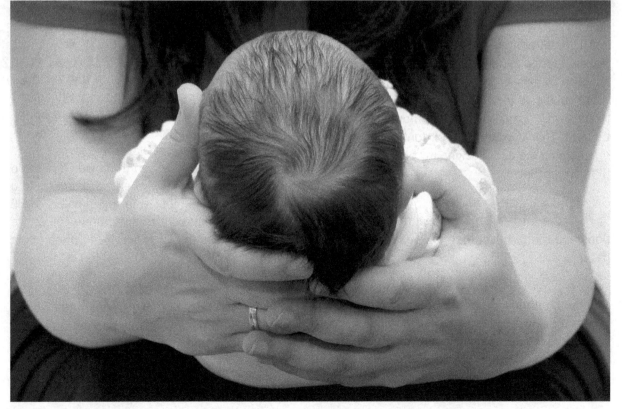

Self-Directed Pregnancy and Birth

Sandra, 41
Job title: Author

1st Child: Girl (3.5 y), freebirth
2nd Child: Boy (1 mo), freebirth

"My whole life, whenever I thought about birth, I imagined doing it by myself."

When I hear the word 'freebirth', the following thoughts pop into my head: A birth that happens alone, in self direction and without anyone in attendance. Consciously chosen and intended, i.e. preplanned or 'by accident' because maybe things happened quickly.

When did you first have the idea to birth without a midwife? When I was 19 or 20. My whole life, whenever I thought about birth, I imagined doing it by myself because I am someone who does better with privacy and the ability to decide things for myself and no observers who might inhibit me.

Who did you tell of your plans? Nobody directly. I didn't dare tell anyone that I felt able to do it myself even for my first birth. And that I think it will go better if no one else is there. I occasionally mentioned to people that I have imagined doing birth by myself. But when comments such as: 'No! You will be pleased when there is someone helping you.' came, I kept my mouth shut and thought: This is exactly what I don't want, someone helping me and blocking my progress, rather than supporting it.

How did the pregnancy go and who did your antenatal care? There were no complications and the birth centre midwives did my antenatal care.

Why did you choose freebirth for yourself? I thought, although I had no previous birth experience that I would be someone for whom maximum privacy was the most important thing during birth. And that I'd be someone who would react with shutting down or shame if someone tried to interfere in the birth.

How did you prepare for the birth? I read lots of books on natural birth, as well as 'Unassisted Childbirth' (Shanley). In pregnancy I did lots of yoga and bellydancing and listened to lots of relaxation cds such as hypnobirthing.

How did the birth go – any complications? Birth happened quickly and only lasted about 2.5 hours from the first contraction. The contractions were more forceful than I imagined which shocked me. But all in all I did well and because my daughter practically shot out of me after 4–5 pushes, there was never the worry that things were not going as they should. My husband insisted I call the midwife a few minutes before birth and I told her I had been having contractions for 2 hours, they were very close together and I already felt like pushing.

The midwife did not take me seriously as I had only been contracting for 2 hours and because I sounded so normal on the phone. She didn't come and just said to call back in a few hours. Although I was outraged she didn't believe me and actually told me I should suppress my urge to push, I was secretly pleased that I was free to do the birth myself. Then I birthed my daughter into my own hands: the most amazing moment of all! Only about 8 minutes after the phone call as we were able to see from our itemised phone bill in retrospect.

How did you experience the postnatal period? My memories of the postnatal period are not all that positive as my sacrum had been brought out of alignment at the birth and I could hardly walk for the pain and wasn't able to carry my daughter initially. That was only possible after a few weeks when my osteopath had treated my sacrum. I have now found out from my midwife that this doesn't necessarily have anything to do with the fast birth (as I had assumed). I also had breastfeeding problems and issues with my midwife who was less than supportive. I eventually found the help I needed from a postnatal doula and La Leche League. At some point we figured breastfeeding out and I am still nursing my 3.5 yo daughter now.

What would you tell other mothers-to-be?

They should ask themselves honestly: Am I someone who needs help (and some people do) or am I someone who deals better with an intimate situation such as birth alone? And then they should follow their gut and not be swayed. Other's advice is generally based on their own lived experience, fears and need for security. But people are very individual in their needs (homebirths always seemed safer to me than hospital births considering the intervention you experience during them) and know themselves well so that they can estimate what is best. Generally I have to say that a pregnant or birthing woman's feelings are a better indicator of how things are going than a thousand machines or other people's opinions.

What would you do differently during another pregnancy and birth?

I found a home-birth midwife for this most recent pregnancy and have not used the birth clinic midwives. I was careful to choose an older midwife who has had children herself (which was not the case with the birth centre midwife). I'm also going to be honest this time, so I told the midwife during our first chat that I may well only call her after the birth. She was ok with that. She just remarked dryly that most women who would rather birth by themselves call too late anyway. She had experienced this a few times already.

Addendum: In May 2014 I birthed our son quickly and without problems – after only 20 minutes and only 4 contractions – at home, alone, only my husband was there. We called the midwife about an hour after birth. I am so thankful I was able to experience 2 lovely, calm, uncomplicated and fast freebirths, that just happened naturally. Births like that are a gift, I think. But they are also normal.

It is probably how births would usually go if women were not so fearful and dramatic.

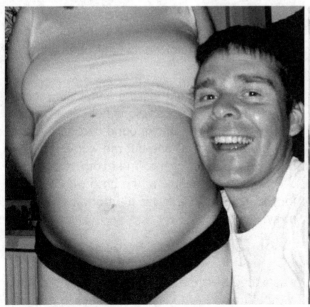

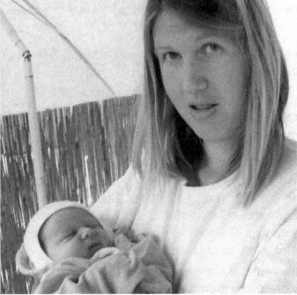

Yvonne, 44
Job title: industrial clerk, full time mother

1st Child: Girl (21 y), hospital birth
2nd Child: Girl (20 y), hospital birth
3rd Child: Boy (5 y), homebirth
4th Child: Boy (3 y), homebirth
5th Child: Girl (1 y), unplanned freebirth

> "I birthed my baby, just like that and without a midwife. Even a year later this puts a smile on my face and makes me feel like I'm walking on air."

When I hear the word 'freebirth', the following thoughts pop into my head: Undisturbed, self determined, good physical awareness. Other people often mention the bravery it requires.

When did you first have the idea to birth without a midwife? It was a bit of an unpleasant thought during the pregnancy as we were having a winter baby. I was a bit worried as my midwife is a good 30 minutes drive away (with clear roads) and I suspected she might not make it in the case of snow and ice (I was due in December). Preparation for the 'worst case scenario' started early with the help of the midwife.

Who did you tell of your plans? Nobody, it just happened that way.

How did the pregnancy go and who did your antenatal care? The pregnancy went well without too much excitement, with midwifery care.

Why did you chose freebirth for yourself? I didn't really think about it until about 5 minutes before the birth.

How did you prepare for the birth? I kept talking through 'What if ...' questions with the midwife. Nothing apart from that.

How did the birth go – any complications? We waited a long time for contractions after my waters went (about 12 hours). Both my sons were born about 2 hours after this happening but my youngest obviously wanted to do things differently and that was unusual to me.

My 'little' daughter (18) and my babysitter (21) were there the whole day, and my husband and sons were there for quite some time too. We laughed, cleaned, cooked and later ate together, the midwife was there in the morning and late afternoon and she went home just after dinner because everything was quiet. The boys were on their way to bed with daddy (upstairs) and I was in the bathroom with the girls. Then suddenly some slightly painful contractions, nothing relevant for birth I thought, no reason to call the midwife – and 50 minutes later my little daughter was born, quietly, relaxed, peaceful and without complications.

Both my birth partners were somewhat speechless, and I was simply overwhelmed – I birthed my baby, just like that and without a midwife. Even a year later this puts a smile on my face and makes me feel like I'm walking on air. Wow!

How did you experience the postnatal period? Exhausting because there were other small and big people mingling about in the house. A bit more peace and quiet would have been great.

What would you tell other mothers-to-be? Informing yourself and asking about the process of birth as early as possible is helpful. A competent midwife in the background can be calming. The thought that no one but me would birth this baby was helpful for me. Trust your body, it can do it. Only have people at the birth who are good for you. If your gut tells you differently, send them away!

What would you do differently during another pregnancy and birth? My fifth pregnancy was altogether great, I would do exactly the same with future children.

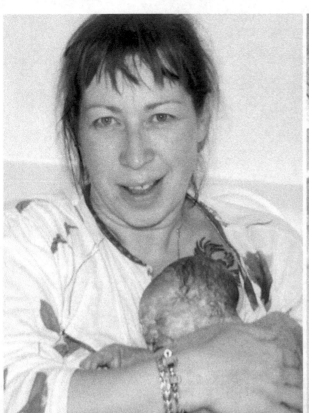
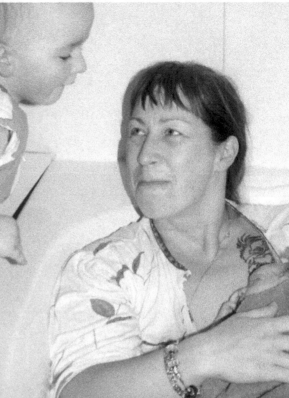

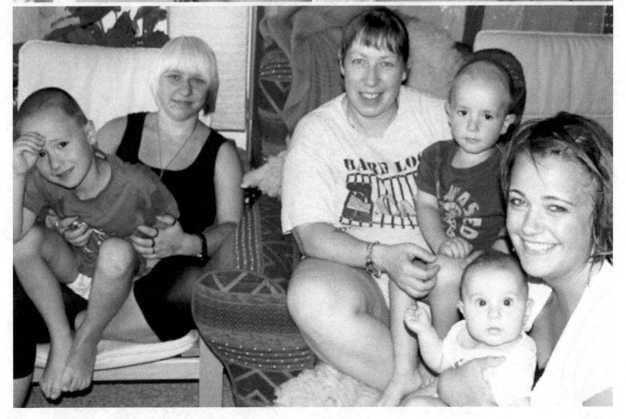

Freebirths with obstacles

Nancy, 27
Job title: Nurse, now full time mother

"The birth was wonderful and easy despite the very big baby."

1st Child: Girl (5 y) hospital birth
2nd Child: Girl (3 y) hospital birth (nearly in the car)
3rd Child: Boy (1 y) freebirth
4th Child: on the way, planned freebirth

When I hear the word 'freebirth', the following thoughts pop into my head: self-directed, without interruptions. No interventions, no 'danger from others' with regards to birth risks.

When did you first have the idea to birth without a midwife? I had the idea quite late really, around the 34th week of pregnancy. It developed 'out of necessity' as the closest midwife lived quite far away and might have been too late for the birth. Over time, the idea sounded better and better to me, until in the end I had a planned birth without attendants.

Who did you tell of your plans? Only my husband.

How did the pregnancy go and who did your antenatal care? The pregnancy was completely normal, apart from apparently having gestational diabetes. I (unfortunately) had a glucose tolerance test and the results were slightly abnormal. So I started checking my blood sugars 3 times daily and when I stopped indulging after 10pm my levels normalised. However, there was unnecessary panic and superfluous tests.

Why did you choose freebirth for yourself? Because I need peace and quiet during birth. It disturbs me when people faff around with me or even inside of me. I don't want to be pulled out of my birth trance and can only let go when I feel undisturbed and safe. To open fully, I need privacy that I can't achieve even with a lovely midwife present.

How did you prepare for the birth? I read a huge amount. Midwifery books as well as videos

have confirmed my wish even more to me. Apart from that I got something to cover the floor and pads for me. I didn't need anything else.

How did the birth go – any complications? The birth was wonderful and easy despite the very big baby. I didn't tear or had any other problems. Because of his size (57 cm long and 4698 g heavy) and the speed of his birth he had a very blue face (congested) and only initiated breathing when I did some mouth to mouth myself.

My husband was unable to judge the situation appropriately and called an ambulance which caused unnecessary medical intervention. They took my son to the neonatal intensive care unit. When I arrived there, he had a gastric tube and was connected to several drips. Despite all tests being normal, they insisted on him having prophylactic antibiotics: 'When you have a homebirth, there are lots of germs about. So we are going to give these until we can prove that there is no infection.'

Because there was no evidence that he needed treatment for anything I decided to take him home. The doctor then told me all sorts of horror stories and remarked how irresponsible I was. Thankfully I was brave enough to take him home the same day, against medical advice.

How did you experience the postnatal period? Due to the trouble we experienced right after the birth, the postnatal period was drenched in tears. Physically, apart from thrush for me and my son, I was fit and well.

What would you tell other mothers-to-be? Don't let others take responsibility for your pregnancy and birth! Birth is NOT a medical process – it is the most natural thing in the world! You can give birth. Have trust!

What would you do differently during another pregnancy and birth? I am currently pregnant and won't see a doctor. My care, only the most necessary bits, will be done by a midwife. Apart from an ultrasound in the 20th week of pregnancy to check for placental location and any abnormalities I will stay away from obstetrics and medical equipment.

I will likely birth all by myself, even without my husband to eliminate any outside fear. After the birth I will call the midwife.

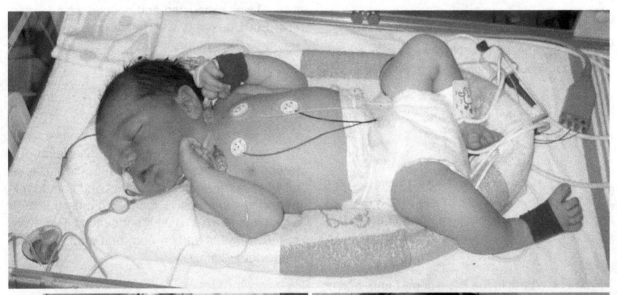

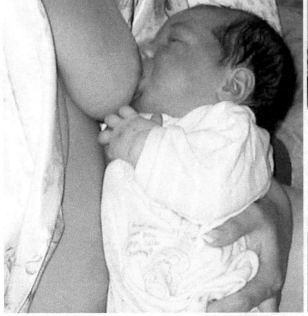

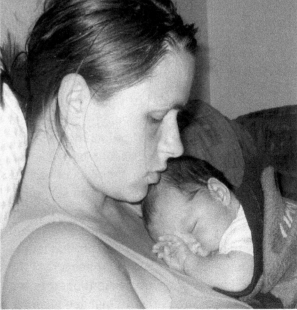

Sarah, 29
Job title: Mother, babywearing consultant

"The most important thing is to listen to yourself and your body."

1st Child: Boy (4.5 y), homebirth
2nd Child: Boy (2 ¾ y), homebirth
3rd Child: Girl (6 mo), homebirth after starting off as freebirth

When I hear the word 'freebirth', the following thoughts pop into my head: Trust in yourself, peaceful, undisturbed.

When did you first have the idea to birth without a midwife? At the beginning of my third pregnancy. The second birth was so lovely and easy, that I could imagine having a freebirth.

Who did you tell of your plans? My husband. He was completely behind me. My midwife was also aware.

How did the pregnancy go and who did your antenatal care? It was a calm, uncomplicated pregnancy. After 35 weeks I started having some productive contractions so I had lots of rest.

Why did you choose freebirth for yourself? I wished for a birth in the circle of my family and no intervention from outsiders.

How did you prepare for the birth? I read a lot, visualised and imagined how it would be. I tried to keep negative thoughts away.

How did the birth go – any complications? Contractions began in the evening – my husband put the older ones to bed. I prepared everything between contractions and lit our birth candle. Quickly contractions got stronger, lots of vocalising and circling my pelvis. My husband supported me, breathing with me. At some point, I just had a weird feeling – the knowledge that I would need help. My midwife was very hands off and let me do what felt good. 1.5 hours after her arrival the baby was born with an asynclitic (tipped to the side) head – placenta after 45 minutes (no intervention) but unfortunately incomplete – manual removal by midwife.

How did you experience the postnatal period? I was exhausted and needed time to process. But I was very well taken care of and was happy to be at home.

What would you tell other mothers-to-be? The most important thing is to listen to yourself and your body.

What would you do differently during another pregnancy and birth? I still dream of a freebirth. The decision to call the midwife after all was right for me in retrospect and I am thankful for her unintrusive manner during the birth and her expertise when it got serious. However I still trust myself and my body and would walk the same path again.

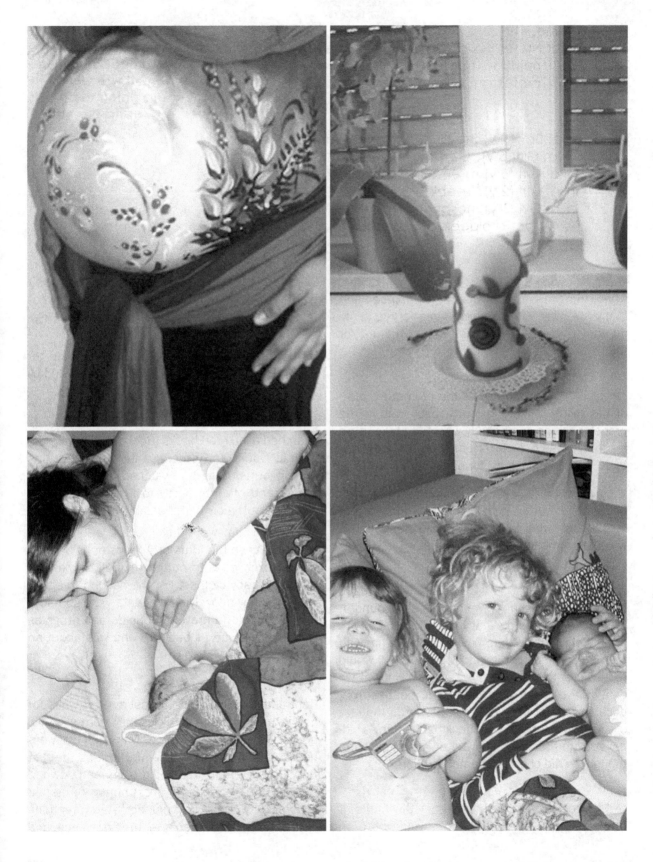

Self-Directed Pregnancy and Birth

Seraphine, 41
Job title: Nurse, educator (food science, nutrition, home economics and protestant religion/theology)

"After the premature birth of the twins, when the fourth baby was in the breech position and nobody wanted to take us on for care, it was definitely clear to us: We are going to do THIS by ourselves, for us and our baby."

1st Child: Boy (9 y), hospital birth with early discharge
2nd Child: Girl (5 y), premature twin birth in the hospital
3rd Child: Girl (5 y), premature twin birth in the hospital
4th Child: Girl (2 y), freebirth
5th Child: Girl (1 y), hospital birth after planned freebirth, caesarean section due to placental abruption with a low lying anterior placenta.

When I hear the word 'freebirth', the following thoughts pop into my head: For me, freebirthing means to birth at my own speed and in my own way, without anyone interfering, thinking they might know what is best for me and/or my child.

When did you first have the idea to birth without a midwife? After the premature birth of the twins, when the fourth baby was in the breech position and nobody wanted to take us on for care, it was definitely clear to us: We are going to do THIS by ourselves, for us and our baby.

Who did you tell of your plans? We were open about the idea but didn't shout it from the roof tops. People who asked got an honest answer: we will allow our child to be born at home.

How did the pregnancy go and who did your antenatal care? Due to the problems in the previous pregnancy, we had an ultrasound at the doctors where our baby was diagnosed with renal pelvis dilatation. When checking in with the paediatric doctor it was clear the baby would require treatment after birth. Apart from that we didn't have much antenatal care, neither from doctor nor midwife – and none towards the end of pregnancy (apart from checking the baby's kidneys). With the fifth child we had even less care, though we did check placental position.

Why did you choose freebirth for yourself? After our first birth with early discharge, it was clear that all other children would be born

at home. Then the twins were born early and we had to go to the hospital. Another birth that didn't go the way I wanted it to. Someone told me what to do constantly: Breathe like this, hold your legs like that, push now ...

Birth is supposed to be something intimate for me and my husband. I don't want to be guided by someone else. So we decided on a freebirth.

How did you prepare for the birth? We researched a lot, read books (Rockenschaub, Hildebrandt, Odent and others) and internet forums (hausgeburtsforum.de), watched videos of freebirths (and others), partly to prepare the other children for the birth of the baby.

Apart from that we didn't prepare a lot: A cord clamp, in case the lotus birth does not work out, some frozen peas to put on my belly in case of bleeding, baby clothes. For the second freebirth with the known low lying placenta we also had a first aid kit with intravenous fluids and drugs as well as a midwife as back up who was about an hour away.

How did the birth go – any complications? Contractions generally only last a short while for my births and the baby is usually born within 6 hours of the first contraction. Transition is always bearable and pushing is painful. During the first freebirth (the fourth baby did turn head down in the end) I experienced a short period of uterine hyperactivity. Our baby did not start breathing spontaneously, not even after the first minute and then turned blue and limp. Massaging her feet and back and blowing in her face didn't work. Only some suction and mouth to mouth resuscitation did eventually work. The cord was very short and I could not put the baby on my chest comfortably. Because the placenta was still in situ even after 2 hours despite strong after pains we decided to cut the cord so I could get into different positions. Using various tricks of the trade the placenta finally came, complete and without pain.

The second freebirth started with the breaking of my waters. Not typical for me as my waters normally go when I push the baby out. About 24 hours after the rupture of membranes the baby turned transverse. It had occasionally taken up this position in pregnancy but could always be persuaded back into a long lie by me lying on my side. In the night after my waters went I lay down on my side again as usual in this situation and put a firm breastfeeding pillow under my bump. Due to the lack of space the baby turned oblique, a lie nearly compatible with vaginal birth.

After my water had been broken for 32 hours without contractions I noticed that something felt different just above my symphysis pubis. The feeling was one of 'something is rummaging around in my belly' and later turned into discomfort. I went to the toilet because I thought I might be losing more liquor (which gets produced constantly, the baby was not 'dry' for 32 hours). This is where I noticed that I was not losing liquor but blood. The bleeding was like a constant thin stream of water. I tried to get dressed but all pads and clothes immediately got soaked so I called the hospital to tell them that I needed to come in and my history as well as informing them that I would need an emergency section and to please get theatre ready. The grandparents were already with the older children and took me and my husband to the hospital. There I was in theatre very quickly, shortly after a vaginal examination. 30 minutes after the bleeding started our baby was born, with collapsed umbilical cord and the need for resuscitation. (Severe asphyxia, Apgars 3/4/6). Immediately before the section the baby had turned back into transverse lie. Our child is now completely healthy and has not sustained any lasting damage.

How did you experience the postnatal period? After the first freebirth: I was fit and well right after the birth and there for my family. I did have excruciating after pains I only managed to cope with taking painkillers. Apart from that we didn't have a calm postnatal period as our baby needed several operations in the first few weeks after birth.

After the abandoned freebirth/caesarean section: our baby recovered amazingly quickly and I discharged myself 48 hours after birth as I didn't want to expose ourselves to unnecessary intervention. Difficulties in this postnatal period were due to my painful fresh caesarean wound as well as my weak general condition due to the severe blood loss.

What would you tell other mothers-to-be? Inform yourself! Birth is all yours. Don't hand it over to someone else. Trust yourself, your body and your child.

What would you do differently during another pregnancy and birth? I suffered a marginal placenta praevia in my pregnancy following my freebirth. Despite that we planned a freebirth, this time with midwives in the background and drugs as back up. However: Another baby will certainly be allowed to be born via freebirth and will likely only experience one detailed ultrasound in pregnancy. I only want midwifery care when I feel it appropriate.

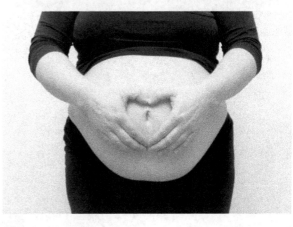

Small and still freebirths

Anna, 25
Job title: Artist and housewife

1st Child: Girl/boy (4 months ago),
small freebirth at 9 weeks pregnant

"At one point I needed the toilet and this is when it came out ... I held it in my hand and said goodbye."

When I hear the word 'freebirth', the following thoughts pop into my head: That birth can be a positive experience.

When did you first have the idea to birth without a midwife? Not at all, it was unplanned.

Who did you tell of your plans? No one, it was unplanned.

How did the pregnancy go and who did your antenatal care? It was only short. Mid November I had a stall at several Christmas markets and was somewhat stressed. At the market before the last one I suddenly realised my period was late by 2 weeks. I went and bought a test and it was positive. I told my boyfriend and we just stood there for quite some time, just laughing and being silly. Seems like we are going to be parents. 'Hahaha' 'You, a dad!' 'And you, a mum!' And just like everyone, I went to the doctor.

I had a scan (I did not feel good and had the feeling I could feel the ultrasound waves), and there was our little worm, I even saw the heartbeat. WOW!

The doctor was odd though and didn't really tell me anything. I asked her if I should be careful with anything. 'No raw meats!' – Ah well, I am vegetarian, I think I can manage that. 'And no smoking and drinking.' Anything else? 'No.'

Ok. So I left the examination room and showed my darling the picture. He was so proud. We were really happy and I just felt complete. Before nothing was amiss but now I was somehow whole.

Why did you choose freebirth for yourself?

In hospital they told me that my baby was still alive, the heart was beating but that I would lose the baby soon. I didn't want to stay there under any circumstances and drove home.

How did you prepare for the birth?

Not at all.

How did the birth go – any complications? One day I had some spotting. The next day I had a scan and everything seemed ok, the baby had grown. We were still happy, a little bit worried, yes ... but I still believed everything would be fine. The bleeding didn't stop. Just a little bit of old blood. A few days later (I can't remember exactly when) there was some fresh blood too. No doctor's surgeries were open so we went to the hospital.

The emergency doctor didn't have a clue. He asked if the baby was moving. No, dearest doctor, in the 8th week of pregnancy you can't generally feel much. Then I was allowed to have a ride in a wheelchair. (I really could have walked but I had always wanted to try so I didn't say anything.)

The doctor checked me and the baby had grown again. I got this injection, as I am rhesus negative. At home my boyfriend explained the scan to me. I was supposed to rest and lie down a lot.

I was not happy about that. I like being active and move about (relatively) frequently. A few days later, a Saturday, I had abdominal pain and bled a fair bit. That's what you get for lying about. Back to the hospital.

The doctor poked me with her instruments for ages, quite brutally too. It hurt and I told her so. No reaction. She did the scan, but so that I could not see the screen.

'Yes. So. The baby is alive. And the heart is beating. BUT not for long.'

'Thanks, I guess I will see myself. I'm sure we'll manage. I'm going home.'

'Well, you'll have to sign something for me.'

I signed her piece of paper, went home and lay down. My love got some food for us and we chatted. At one point I needed the toilet and this is when it came out. I didn't want it to be true. There was the amniotic sac and everything. I held it in my hand and said goodbye. We buried our baby in my step father's garden.

How did you experience the postnatal period? I cried and screamed the whole night. I blamed myself and cursed everyone and everything. My mother said I needed to go to the doctor's again. I didn't want to but gave in. So I went to the clinic that Monday.

The nurse looked at my notes and looked at my scan pictures. 'Oh, it is you! Wait here please.' Half an hour later I was still sitting there although they told me to come IMMEDIATELY on the phone.

So I went to the nurse and asked her why it was taking that long. 'Well, listen, you are not the only one here! We had to squeeze you in and there are a couple of people before you!'

I was close to crying. I want to go! 'I do not recommend that!'

I will go now. Run towards the exit. 'You'll have to sign something!'

Took piece of paper and pen. I'M GOING NOW! *signed* Stormed out. I cried and screamed the whole way home.

The following weeks were pretty awful. My family didn't understand. 'That was nothing, it was so very little. At 9 weeks it's not really a person yet.'

I was advised to stay in bed to rest, but I didn't want to. I went on a long shopping trip with my love and my best friend.

My friend drove 500km to be with me and the week after we spent drinking and gambling. Physically I was fine after that.

I had a period for about a week and the next couple of periods were somewhat heavier than normal. I have not been to a doctor since.

What would you tell other mothers-to-be? Decline ultrasounds and unnecessary examinations! Doctors only make you and your baby feel insecure.

What would you do differently during another pregnancy and birth? Not going to the doctor. No ultrasounds.

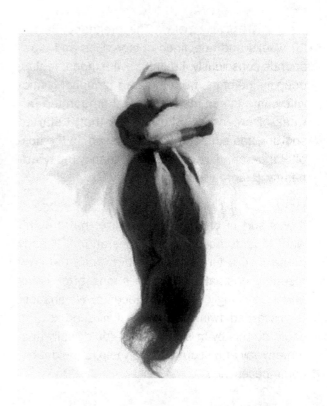

Katharina, 28
Job title: Mother and student

"Apart from a lot of chocolate for the soul I didn't really prepare anything."

1st Child: Girl (4 y) hospital birth
2nd Child: Girl (2 y) homebirth
3rd Child: Boy/Girl (about 1.5 years ago) small freebirth in 10th week of pregnancy

When I hear the word 'freebirth', the following thoughts pop into my head: The ability to trust in one's body, calm, self determination, unleashing your primal power.

When did you first have the idea to birth without a midwife? Just briefly during my second pregnancy, but really I didn't think it was my 'thing'. I thought about it a lot more before and during my miscarriage. Now, after, I can imagine having a happy freebirth.

Who did you tell of your plans? No one knew I was pregnant, only my husband and midwife. It was clear to both of them I would try to do it at home.

How did the pregnancy go and who did your antenatal care? The pregnancy lasted 10 weeks and I declined doctor visits and ultrasounds consciously. I didn't have a 'good' feeling deep inside of me from the start though. My midwife came to see me for the first time in the 9th week of pregnancy. Shortly after that, I started spotting and suddenly wanted a scan. In the hospital they found a non viable pregnancy (no heartbeat and far too small).

Why did you choose freebirth for yourself? It was sort of obvious I'd try it like that. I didn't want to go to hospital for an operation. I already had a D&C after the second birth (due to heavy bleeding postnatally despite strong after pains and a seemingly complete placenta. We suspect a miscarried twin.) I felt that I needed to and could do this by myself. No one could really help me anyway and I could call for help, should it become necessary.

How did you prepare for the birth? Not really at all. I had read reports of miscarriages, but never imagined it to be like this. I knew it would just start at some point. Apart from a lot of chocolate for the soul I didn't really prepare anything.

How did the birth go – any complications? I felt it went ok. The bleeding increased, and strong and painful contractions started. I took a small bowl, put it between my legs and leaned over the sofa on all fours bleeding into it. Blood flowed after every contraction, but not in waves. It seemed to come out as bigger clots. I couldn't see any actual fetal tissue.

After about 3 hours it was over and the bleeding continued like a period. The next morning some tissue came out. It looked like placenta. As a layperson I estimate that I lost about 500 ml of blood in the three hours of labour. I never felt faint.

How did you experience the postnatal period? I was surprised that I definitely felt 'postnatal' after the miscarriage. I didn't know it could be like that after an early miscarriage. I was happy and a little hyper that I managed it myself, the same hormonal high like after a 'proper' birth.

After that I became sad again, but not as sad as I thought I might be. The bleeding became less and less. A few days after the miscarriage I lost another bigger chunk of tissue. After that the bleeding reduced even more until there was only some brown spotting left. This stopped after a few more days.

What would you tell other mothers-to-be? You can of course have a D&C but the female body manages miscarriages beautifully by itself.

I'm sure in most cases this is much better for your hormone levels and your soul. These days we paint a very disjointed picture of miscarriage and its potential complications. The risks of a D&C are very much understated.

What would you do differently during another pregnancy and birth? I would do exactly the same. Everything was as it was supposed to be.

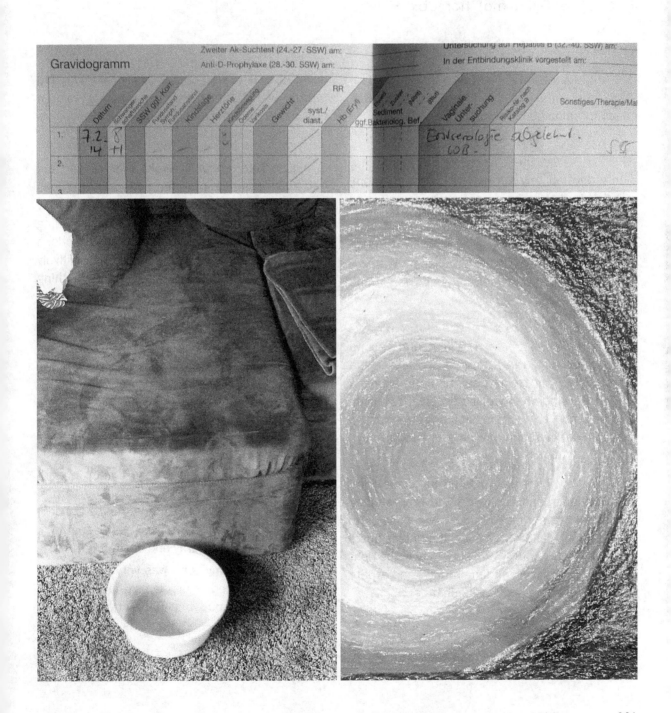

Marina, 32
Job title: teacher for German as a foreign language, translator

"My doctor recommended to just go home and wait for nature to take its course."

1st Child: Girl/Boy (5.5 years ago), small freebirth
2nd Child: Girl/Boy (5 years ago), small freebirth
3rd Child: Boy (3 y), hospital birth (ventouse)
4th Child: Girl (6 mo), homebirth

When I hear the word 'freebirth', the following thoughts pop into my head: Self determined, normal, free, natural.

When did you first have the idea to birth without a midwife? When my first pregnancy didn't develop any further, my doctor recommended to just go home and wait for nature to take its course.

Who did you tell of your plans? Pretty much everyone who knew of the pregnancy. With my first miscarriage that was nearly all friends and family, with the second only a few.

How did the pregnancy go and who did your antenatal care? The first and second pregnancies ended in a missed abortion and a 'small birth'. The third was an unproblematic pregnancy under the care of a doctor. The fourth: no problems, care from my doctor in the first trimester, after that from a wonderful midwife.

Why did you choose freebirth for yourself? The first time because I trusted my doctor and her experience and because I had read studies that showed this course of action was quite safe. I also did not want to go to hospital unless absolutely necessary. Intuitively I knew it was the right path for me. The second time round I had experience and knew my body could do it.

How did you prepare for the birth? I read studies on 'Expectant management of missed abortion', chatted with women who had experienced similar situations (in forums), prayed and used the time to say goodbye to my baby who had passed away. Before the birth of my living children I read a lot about active physiological birth.

How did the birth go – any complications?
1. miscarriage: about 4 weeks after diagnosis I had a few days of painful contractions, sometimes close together sometimes far apart. On the day of the actual miscarriage I worked in the morning then suddenly had strong relentless contractions when I got home and heavy bleeding. Intuitively I had a bath, and a few minutes later everything came out and the bleeding stopped.

2. miscarriage: nearly the same, but a bit faster, again in the bath. No complications.

My son was born by ventouse in the hospital. My daughter was born at home, completely relaxed. I knew exactly what I needed at all times during that birth and was sure she was well.

How did you experience the postnatal period? After the first miscarriage I went to work the next day as normal (a half day). The second miscarriage happened on Christmas eve and I was off work for about two weeks after that, so I could lie down, rest plenty and cry it out.

After the birth of my son I was very stressed because of breastfeeding problems (thankfully overcome now), but proud and happy. After my daughter's birth I enjoyed every single day.

What would you tell other mothers-to-be? Trust your body and listen to your intuition.

What would you do differently during another pregnancy and birth? For the birth of my son I went to hospital because I was naive enough to hope for a natural and intervention free birth. I experienced the birth of my daughter as free and self determined, my midwife came for the pushing phase. Should I have another baby, I know I would be able to give birth to it without help. During birth I know best if and when support is needed.

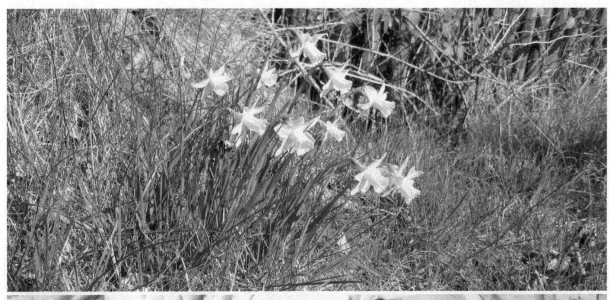

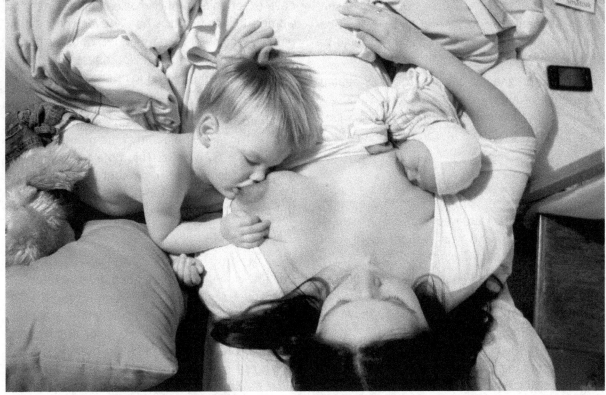

Annalies, 39
Job title: project manager, advisor

1st Child: Boy (6 y), premature birth (36 weeks) in
    an anthroposophical hospital
2nd Child: Girl/Boy (4 years ago), small freebirth in 13th week
    of pregnancyChild: Boy (2 y) hospital birth in
    an anthroposophical hospital (felt like a freebirth
    with husband and midwife in the background)

"Giving birth in dignity is an empowering experience for a woman, and its influence on a self determined life (and the life of the child) should not be underestimated."

When I hear the word 'freebirth', the following thoughts pop into my head: The word 'freebirth' makes me think of peace, a complete being within myself, and mastering the birth 'alone', self determined. Freebirth means feeling a strong sense of strength, dignity, and trust in the process.

When did you first have the idea to birth without a midwife? When I found out that I was going to have a miscarriage at nine weeks pregnant, I wanted to stay in control.

Who did you tell of your plans? After consulting my husband, my doctor and my midwife it became clear that a small birth at home would be my/our path – as long as it felt safe.

In my third pregnancy, convinced by my healing experience of miscarriage I wanted to work with the natural process myself. I made a wish list I gave to the staff in the (anthroposophical) hospital.

How did the pregnancy go and who did your antenatal care? The second pregnancy went well initially. I enjoyed the strong nausea and achy breasts and was excited about mine and my husband's little secret.

Interestingly I did think about an early end to this pregnancy now and again. Two of my friends had just experienced 3 miscarriages and I think this was why the thought came up. In the 9th week of pregnancy I went to get my official notes so I could sort out the official paperwork with my employer and insurance. The scan at the doctors showed there was no heartbeat and the baby's growth did not correspond to 9 weeks gestation. The doctor was sensitive and wanted to book me in for a D&C for the following day. Sad and overwhelmed I declined and we decided to wait another week. I contacted our midwife and we talked. It became clear there was no rush as long as I was well. After one, then two weeks had passed, my doctor became more and more nervous and started quoting textbooks, but did actually understand where I was coming from. I think highly of her as she admitted she simply does not have experience in physiological miscarriages as women in her practice hardly ever choose that path. My midwife recommended another doctor experienced in 'natural miscarriage'. She had a chat with me and offered to be there for me in an emergency or in the case I changed my mind.

My third pregnancy was unremarkable apart from pelvic girdle pain and some premature contractions at 32 weeks. This time I was not worried about losing this little soul before its time. My midwife did my antenatal care. I only went to the doctor to diagnose the pregnancy and for 3 scans.

Why did you choose freebirth for yourself? Our first son's birth happened without intervention, at least until I held him in my arms. We were however transferred to a clinic with a neonatal unit after his birth at 35 +5 – for observation. There, we really had to fight to make decisions about our son's health care. It quickly became clear he was completely healthy, yet they did not want to discharge him. He was small and light, completely normal for the 36th week of gestation. My milk didn't come in, not surprisingly considering the scary situation we were in, coupled with the anger and grief regarding the loss of my peaceful postnatal period.

The protocols in the hospital were very much determined by blood tests and machinery, and the obvious development of the baby (as well as maternal gut feeling) were very much overlooked. I needed a week to get back into control and organise our discharge. I found myself hurt and, retrospectively, psychologically traumatised in this sensitive phase after the birth of my first child.

In the months after the birth, our midwife was my biggest support and most enduring listening ear. The experience has taught me how important making my own decisions is for my spiritual health.

The midwife was my first port of call when I found out about the impending miscarriage in my second pregnancy. When I was told that complications would be unlikely as long as I felt healthy and the risk of infection would be similar to after a D&C in the hospital, it was clear to me that I wanted to let nature take its course. I went into myself a lot in that time – I still had strong pregnancy symptoms. I was sure I could trust my body and the time for miscarriage had not quite come yet. An intensive period of saying goodbye followed, in a spiritual and physical sense.

In my third pregnancy, this experience turned out to be my anchor. I had the feeling all would be well if I could make my own decisions.

How did you prepare for the birth? After consulting my doctor and midwife, a phase of intensive inner reflection followed. I read a lot and drew strength from 'normal' homebirth stories on the internet.

I felt my loss and grieved. Interestingly, I got the time for that because saying goodbye took about 4 weeks. My midwife gave me advice about what I could do for worries and heavy bleeding with herbal teas and homeopathy. Then came the waiting and observing how my body very slowly turned 'unpregnant'. I could practically feel how my pregnancy hormone levels dropped and the end of pregnancy got closer and closer.

The third pregnancy was marked by trust in my body and the feeling 'I can manage/I can do it.' Again, I read a lot of homebirth and freebirth stories on the internet. Those gave me peace and trust. I thank all those women who made their stories and videos available online!

I thought carefully about what I wanted, and put together the already mentioned wish list. I wanted to be left in peace until I asked for help. And I wanted to be the first to touch the baby.

Why didn't I stay at home? My husband is a doctor (not an obstetrician). He did his obstetric rotation at the university hospital – and has seen all the rare complications you see there. He wanted to be present at the birth without feeling any medical responsibility. And I wanted him present as my husband. The anthroposophical hospital was therefore the best solution for us as a couple.

How did the birth go – any complications? The miscarriage already began 3 weeks before the actual miscarriage with the reduction in pregnancy symptoms. I am very thankful I didn't find out about the miscarriage in hospital with the shock of heavy bleeding as some of my friends had. It gave me room to decide calmly for myself.

About 2 days before the birth I started spotting. I cancelled an impending work trip, called in sick and waited.

Unfortunately I woke with contractions on the night before my husband's birthday at around 2am. I took a book (randomly Turgenjew's 'Fathers and Sons'), snuggled down with my robe and sorted the bathroom. My boys were fast asleep. I could completely focus on the process.

The contractions were regular. I breathed through them. My thoughts were scattered between my body and Turgenjew.

Fairly strong bleeding started with a few biggish blood clots. After about 2-3 hours I passed the amniotic sac with the beginnings of placenta – as far as I could see – and a little structure surrounded by 'roots' (vessels). Once the contractions stopped, normal menstrual bleeding started. I felt closure. Everything was ok as it was. The grief felt less strong. It felt good, like the labour was the last rites.

I think I had the same hormonal response as after birth. I showered, pampered myself and felt powerful. In this mood I suddenly realised how lovely it was that it happened to be my husbands birthday today. I had already prepared for it (as I didn't know the miscarriage would happen tonight) and baked a big batch of buttermilk scones for my love. He had been to university in the US a few years ago and hadn't had scones for ages. So we celebrated 'birth' at breakfast – with an extra little candle on the table.

At the end of my third pregnancy my son's birth went beautifully. After about 3 hours of labour, 25 minutes of that in the hospital, I was the first to touch him. The attending midwife granted all my wishes and didn't do a thing ... apart from providing a dark room with candle light and putting a mat under my knees.

How did you experience the postnatal period? After the miscarriage I rested in bed for a about a day, reflecting on the experience and – this might sound odd, but – happy. I had managed by myself. All in all a very healing experience. A medical check up a few days later proved my physical awareness and showed that my cycle was already continuing as it should.

In the postnatal period with my youngest son I kept asking 'where the catch was'. Everything was practically perfect. We did skin to skin for 2 ½ days, until he put on his very first vest. Until the 10th day I was looked after at home before I was back to everyday life. My family ensured that the little one hardly had to leave our house for the first 13 (!) weeks and could have a very relaxed start in life.

What would you tell other mothers-to-be? Take your gut feeling seriously, even when you are pregnant for the first time! Plan for emergency scenarios. Then put them away in a mental drawer! You can do it! And: Giving birth in dignity is an empowering experience for a woman, and its influence on a self determined life (and the life of the child) should not be underestimated!

What would you do differently during another pregnancy and birth? I would stay at home for birth after a full term pregnancy this time. I think, we are at that point as a family now.

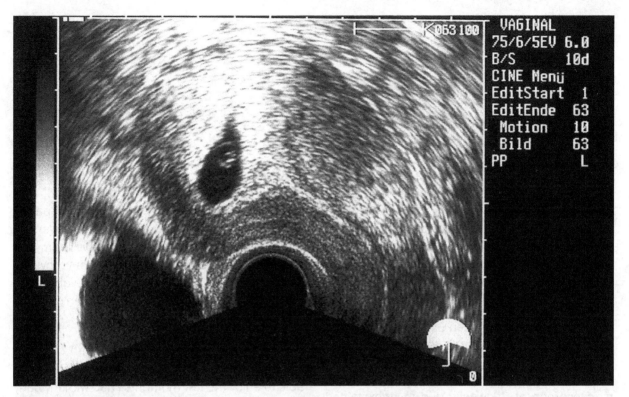

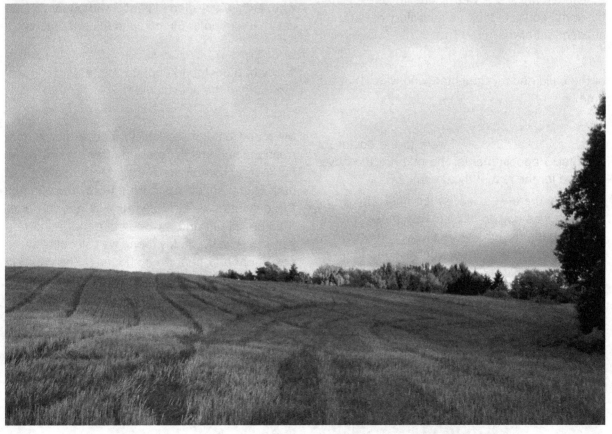

Kerstin, 48
Job title: paediatric nurse

"I asked a friend, a doctor, to support me, and then I surrendered to the unavoidable."

1st Child: Boy (23 y), premature birth in hospital, caesarean
2nd Child: Girl (16 y), homebirth
3rd Child: Boy (6 years ago), still freebirth in the 27th week of pregnancy

When I hear the word 'freebirth', the following thoughts pop into my head: Plenty of knowledge about the natural process of birth, trust in your own physical and spiritual awareness, being secure in yourself and being joyous about the impending miracle ...

When did you first have the idea to birth without a midwife? Even as a young girl I felt a deep 'knowledge and trust' in my ability to give birth as a woman – unfortunately things went very differently with my first child (he was born by caesarean at 29 weeks due to unexplained bleeding) so that I took up midwifery care for my subsequent births.

Who did you tell of your plans? The father of the child and my daughter (who was 10 at the time).

How did the pregnancy go and who did your antenatal care? I went to the doctor for the first 3 appointments, the midwife took over my care for the rest of the pregnancy.

Physically there were no issues until 22 weeks, though I was psychologically very tense (professionally and privately) which showed in occasionally very strong premature contractions from 23 weeks onwards. One evening in the beginning of the 27th week of pregnancy the midwife was unable to pick up the fetal heart. She left our house in a panic. She seemed completely out of her depth and left me in a state of shock.

The next day she took me to a doctor she knew, who confirmed her findings. I didn't want to give birth in the hospital and the midwife said she felt confident attending the birth at home. The doctor was comfortable with this. If my friend, who is a doctor, hadn't come to see me from Spain, I wouldn't have wanted to have any dealings with that midwife anymore and would have let myself go. I was completely separate from my physical self at that point. The pain was unbelievably huge and a part of me died with the baby. An 'I' didn't really exist at that point.

Why did you choose freebirth for yourself? I wanted the security of my own home and to be able to enjoy the few moments I had with my baby who had already died in peace, without any medical intervention or direction, in full awareness.

How did you prepare for the birth? I asked a friend, a doctor, to support me, and then I surrendered to the unavoidable.

How did the birth go – any complications? My friend brought tablets to induce me as contractions had still not started after 3 days. Three hours after contractions finally started, after 2–3 pushes my angel was born into my own hands. But only after we sent the midwife and father of the baby home and my daughter and friend had gone for a lie down. My friend was sleeping in the next room and heard me shouting. She came in right after the birth with my 10 year old daughter. We phoned the midwife for the placenta. No complications.

How did you experience the postnatal period? Deep in grief.

I suppressed lactation by binding my breasts and with homeopathic remedies. I held my son in my arms until the day of his funeral, three days later,

Rose Monday, and therefore also declined a post mortem. I put him into a specially designed coffin with my own hands and put him into my mother's grave to join her. The child seemed completely healthy on the outside, yet very small. However my previous babies had also been small.

One half of the placenta looked thrombosed and partly necrotic. Later I was diagnosed with Factor V Leiden (a hereditary genetic abnormality which predisposes to blood clots). Perhaps this is why the placenta was thrombosed.

I wanted to die after the birth/funeral, the pain was just too much to bear. I didn't eat or drink ANYTHING other than half a glass of orange juice a day for weeks, didn't sleep at all (!) for weeks and stayed on the sofa crying, in front of the snowy television screen. The result: 4 weeks later I had a pulmonary embolus, a deep vein thrombosis in my leg in three spots and went into intensive care (where they diagnosed Factor V Leiden). Two children were at home, no one cared. And to top it all: Noro outbreak on the ward, no visitors for several days – apparently no one available to look after my children, as there were no staff free to do so. I wanted to go HOME to my living children, they needed me!

Ten days later I was discharged, still bedbound, against medical advice.

My little, grown up, wonderful daughter ran the household over the next few weeks until I was able to walk again.

What would you tell other mothers-to-be? A pregnancy and birth is the most wonderful event a woman is able to experience – our healthy body is made to birth babies, and even knows how to deal with stillbirths. Have trust! My last words are the conclusion to my whole experience: I went through hell but learned to see heaven. Only love is eternal. Always. Love IS :-)

What would you do differently during another pregnancy and birth? I would take more care of my own spiritual balance. I would keep visits to the doctor to an absolute minimum.

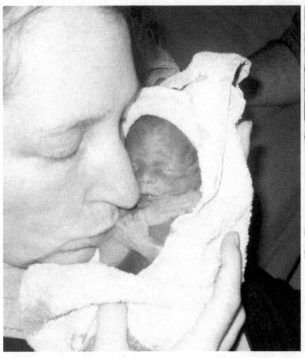
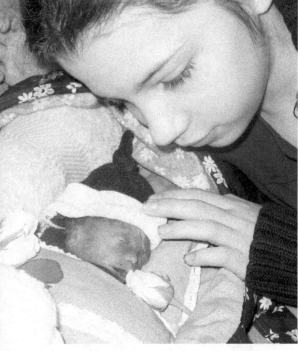

Self-Directed Pregnancy and Birth

Appendix

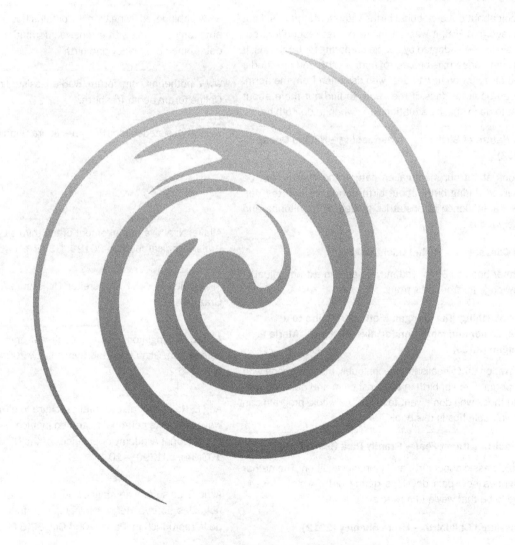

Recommended reading

Understanding and Teaching Optimal Fetal Positioning – Jean Sutton (1996)

A book on getting the baby into the optimal position before birth: this book offers valuable tips and background knowledge.

Ina May's Guide to Childbirth – Ina May Gaskin (2003)

A classic that looks closely at usual hospital routines and encourages self-directed birth with lovely homebirth stories.

Emergency Childbirth – Gregory J. White (1998)

A book about out of hospital births without attendants. First released in 1958, it was originally for first responders but has since been adopted by people preparing for freebirths. It has summarised the process of normal birth and provided a good overview on how to deal with deviation from the norm. A good book for dads, if they want to find out more about what to do in specific situations and when to do nothing.

The Nature of Birth and Breastfeeding – Michel Odent (1992)

A book about our mammalian nature, the need to not be observed during birth, about birth hormones and the detrimental influence of obstetrics guided by monitoring and observations.

The Caesarean – Michel Odent (2004)

Another book by Odent you may be able to extract valuable knowledge for freebirths from.

Hypnobirthing: The Mongan Method: A Guide to a Safe, Easier and more Comfortable Birthing – Marie F. Mongan (2013)

Relaxation and visualisation techniques, that help cope with the primal force of birth in the most calm and painless way. Even those who don't want to follow the whole program can find valuable tips in this book.

Childbirth without Fear – Grantly Dick-Read (2013)

An old classic about birth and pain, new edition. The author describes how pain develops during birth, why it doesn't have to be that way and how to avoid pain.

Unassisted Childbirth – Laura Shanley (2012)

This book is by the American pioneer in all things freebirth. I would have liked to see less personal philosophy and more practical tips. It contains birth stories and thoughts on birth, but is not a handbook for freebirth as such.

These books are ones I have read myself and recommend – apart from the limitations mentioned above. There are lots more helpful books on the market and in the last few years even a few books on freebirths have appeared. I have read some of them, and while the birth stories, thoughts and resulting knowledge are certainly interesting, the obstetric information in those books is not always accurate or well researched.

Further websites

www.unhindered-living.com – Contains tips about autonomous living with extensive information regarding self determined pregnancy and birth.

www.mothering.com/forum/306-unassisted-childbirth – Online forum about freebirth.

www.unassistedchildbirth.com – Laura Shanley's website.

Sources

Aflaifel N: Active management of the third stage of labour. British Medical Journal, 2012 Jul, 345, p. e4546.

Aigelsreiter H: Die 7 Aigelsreiter. Dr. Helmut Aigelsreiter, Graz, 2012.

Alarab M: Singleton vaginal breech delivery at term: still a safe option. Obstetrics and Gynecology, 2004 Mar, 103(3), p. 407–12.

Ang E, Rakic P et al: Prenatal exposure to ultrasound waves impacts neuronal migration in mice. Proceedings of the National Academy of Sciences of the USA, 2006 Aug, 103(34), p. 12903–10.

Azria E: Le sulfate de magnésium en obstétrique : données actuelles. Journal de gynécologie, obstétrique et biologie de la reproduction, Paris, 2004 Oct, 33(6 Pt 1), p. 510–7.

Balki M: Labor-augmenting drug may contribute to reduced effect in controlling postpartum bleeding. American Society of Anesthesiologists, 2013 Aug, 119(3), p. 552.

Barrett L: Birth Video Of A Breech Baby. http://www.homebirth.net.au/2008/04/breech-birth.html, 2008 Apr 16. (abgerufen am 14.5.2014)

Bauer I: Diaper Free: The Gentle Wisdom of Natural Infant Hygiene, Plume, New York City (USA), 2006.

Bauer N: Das Versorgungskonzept Hebammenkreißsaal und die möglichen Auswirkungen auf Gesundheit und Wohlbefinden von Mutter und Kind. Dissertation an der Hochschule für Gesundheit, Bochum, 2011.

Beech B & Robinson J: Ultrasound? Unsound. Association for Improvements in the Maternity Services (AIMS), London, 1996.

Bercik P: The Intestinal Microbiota Affect Central Levels of Brain-Derived Neurotropic Factor and Behavior in Mice. Gatroenterology, 2011 Aug, 141(2), p. 599–609.e1–3.

Berglas A: Cancer: Nature, Cause and Cure. Paris, 1957.

Bergsjö P et al: Duration of human singleton pregnancy. A population-based study. Acta obstetricia et gynecologica Scandinavia, 1990 Jan, 69(3), p. 197–207.

Beuker JM: Is endomyometrial injury during termination of pregnancy or curettage following miscarriage the precursor to placenta accreta? Journal of Clinical Pathology, 2005 Mar, 58(3), p.273–5.

Bouke L: Infant Potty Training: A Gentle and Primeval Method Adapted to Modern Living, White-Boucke Publishing, Lafayette (USA), 2008.

Bowman K: Alignment Matters: The First Five Years of Katy Says. Propriometrics Press, Carlsborg, Washington (USA), 2013.

Boyle JJ, Katz VL: Umbilical cord prolapse in current obstetric practice. Journal of Reproductive Medicine 2005, 50, p. 303–6.

Brocklehurst P: Perinatal and maternal outcomes by planned place of birth for healthy women with low risk pregnancies: the Birthplace in England national prospective cohort study. British Medical Journal, 2011 Nov 25, 343, p. d7400.

Brown K: Diet-Induced Dysbiosis of the Intestinal Microbiota and the Effects on Immunity and Disease. Nutrients, 2012 Oct 26, 4(11), p. 1552.

Campbell JD et al: Case-control study of prenatal ultrasonography exposure in children with delayed speech. Canadian Medical Association Journal, 1993 Nov, 149(10), p. 1435–40.

Caviness VS, Grant PE: Our unborn children at risk? Proceedings of the National Academy of Sciences of the USA, 2006 Aug, 103(34), p. 12661–2.

Chan FY: Limitations of Ultrasound. Paper presented at Perinatal Society of Australia and New Zealand 1st Annual Congress, Freemantle, 1997.

Chauhan SP: Maternal and perinatal complications with uterine rupture in 142,075 patients who attempted vaginal birth after cesarean delivery: A review of the literature. American Journal of Obstetrics and Gynecology, 2003 Aug, 189(2), p. 408–17.

Chervenak FA, McCullough LB: Research on the fetus using Doppler ultrasound in the first trimester: guiding ethical considerations. Ultrasound in Obstetrics and Gynecology, 1999 Sep, 14(3), p. 161.

Clark D: Herbs for Mother's Care Postpartum. Birth Kit, 2004 Winter, p. 44.

Conde-Aqudelo A: Birth Spacing and Risk of Adverse Perinatal Outcomes: a meta-analysis. Journal of the American Medical Association, 2006 Apr 19, 295(15), p. 1809–23.

Corteville JE: Fetal Pyelectasis and Down Syndrome: Is Genetic Amniocentesis Warranted? Obstetrics & Gynecology, 1992 May, 79(5 (Pt 1)), p. 770–2.

Cunningham F, Williams J: Williams Obstetrics, 20th Edition. Appelton & Lange, Stamfort CT USA, 1997, p. 982–7.

Czeizel AE: Folate Deficiency and Folic Acid Supplementation: The Prevention of Neural-Tube Defects and Congenital Heart Defects. Nutrients, 2013 Nov, 5(11), p. 4760–75.

Dahle LO: The effect of oral magnesium substitution on pregnancy-induced leg cramps. American Journal of Obstetric & Gynecology, 1995 Jul, 173(1), p. 175–80.

Davies JA et al: Randomised controlled trial of doppler ultrasound screening of placental perfusion during pregnancy. The Lancet, 1992 Nov, 340(8831), p. 1299–303.

Davis A: Let's have healthy children. New American Library, New York City, 1972.

Debby A: Clinical significance of the floating fetal head in nulliparous women in labor. Journal of Reproductive Medicine, 2003 Jan, 48(1), p. 37–40.

De Tayrac R: Épisiotomie et prévention des lésions pelvi-périnéales. Journal de gynécologie, obstétrique et biologie de la reproduction, Paris, 2006 Feb, 35(1 Suppl), p. 1S24–31.

Dror DK: Effect of vitamin B12 deficiency on neurodevelopment in infants: current knowledge and possible mechanisms. Nutrition reviews, 2008 May, 66(5), p. 250–5.

El Harta V: Posterior Labor: a pain in the back. Midwifery Today, Winter 1995, 36, p. 19–21.

Eirich M, Oblasser C: Luxus Privatgeburt. edition riedenburg, Salzburg 2012.

Erikson S: Vortrag „Ultraschall und Kulturen des Risikos". Tagung „Da stimmt doch was nicht – Logik, Praxis und Folgen vorgeburtlicher Diagnostik", 1. März 2008, Dresden.

Ewigman BG, Crane JP, Frigoletto FD et al: Effect of Prenatal Ultrasound Screeening on Perinatal Outcome, RADIUS Study Group. New England Journal of Medicine, 1993 Sep, 329, p. 821–827.

Ezra Y: Randomized Control Trial for the Comparison of Biologic Glue Versus Suturing for First Degree Perineal Tears. ClinicalTrials.gov NCT00746707, 2014 Mar.

Fischer R: Breech Presentation. www.medscape.org, 2012 Jul 9. (abgerufen am 27.3.2014)

Frimmel TAE: Verbessert sich die Gewichtsschätzung mit Ultraschall durch Einbeziehung der mütterlichen Größe? Dissertation, Technische Universität München Okt 2004.

Gaskin IM, Brunner JP: All-Fours Maneuver for Reducing Shoulder Dystocia During Labor. Journal if Reproductive Medicine, 1998 May, 43, p. 439–43.

Gielchinsky Y: Placenta Accreta – Summary of 10 Years: A Survey of 310 Cases. Placenta, 23(2–3), 2002 Feb, p. 210–4.

Glezerman M: Five years to the term breech trial: the rise and fall of a randomized controlled trial. American Journal of Obstetrics and Gynecology, 2006 Jan, 194(1), p. 20–5.

Goffinet F: Is planned vaginal delivery for breech presentation at term still an option? Results of an observational prospective survey in France and Belgium. American Journal of Obstetrics and Gynecology, 2006 Apr, 194(4), p. 1002–11.

Graf F: Kritik der Arzneiroutine bei Schwangeren und Kleinkindern. Spangsrade Verlag, Ascheberg, 2010.

Greene D: Efficacy of Octyl-2-Cyanoacrylate Tissue Glue in Blepharoplasty: A Prospective Controlled Study of Wound-Healing Characteristics. Archives of Facial Plastic Surgery, 1999 Oct, 1(4), p. 292–6.

Gurven M, Kaplan H: Longevity Among Hunter-Gatherers: A Cross-Cultural Examination. Population and Development Review, 2007 Jun, 33(2), p. 321–65.

Hannah ME: Planned caesarean section versus planned vaginal birth for breech presentation at term: a randomised multicentre trial. Term Breech Trial Collaborative Group. Lancet, 2000 Oct 21, 356(9239), p. 1375–83.

Hartmann K, Viswanathan M: Outcomes of routine episiotomy: a systematic review. Journal of the American Medical Association, 2005 May 4, 293(17), p. 2141–8.

Herrmann W, Obeid R: Ursachen und frühzeitige Diagnostik von Vitamin-B12-Mangel. Deutsches Ärzteblatt, Okt 2008, 105(40), S. 680-5. (Online verfügbar unter: http://www.aerzteblatt.de/pdf.asp?id=61696. Zuletzt geprüft am: 04.04.2014.)

Hessel L: Mothering's UC Roll Call. In: Freeze R: Born free. Unassisted childbirth in North America. Dissertation , University of Iowa (USA) 2008, p. 219.

Hickok DE: The frequency of breech presentation by gestational age at birth: A large population-based study. American Journal of Obstetrics and Gynecology, 1992 Mar, 166(3), p. 851–2.

Hildebrandt S: Nachgeburtsperiode: Zurückhaltung. Deutsche Hebammenzeitschrift, Dez 2008, S. 22–5.

Hogan MC: Maternal mortality for 181 countries, 1980–2008: a systematic analysis of progress towards Millennium Development Goal 5. Lancet, 2010 May, 375(9726), p. 1609–23.

Huber AM, Gershoff SN: Effects of Dietary Zinc and Calcium on the Retention and Distribution of Zinc in Rats Fed Semipurified Diets. Journal of Nutrition, 1970 Aug, 100(8), p. 949–54.

Ijaz N: Unpasteurized milk: myth and evidence. Grand Rounds Presentation BC Centre for Disease Control, 2013 May 13.

Jacques SM : Placenta accreta: mild cases diagnosed by placental examination. International Journal of Gynecological Pathology 1996 Jan, 15, p. 28–33

J-Orh R: Prevalence and associate factors for striae gravidarum. Journal of the Medical Association of Thailand, 2008 Apr, 91(4), p. 445–51.

Jouppila P: Postpartum Haemorrhage. Current Opinion in Obstetric & Gynecology, 1995 Dec, 7(6), p. 446–50.

Jukic AM: Length of human pregnancy and contributors to its natural variation. Journal of Human Reproduction, 2013 Oct, 28(10), p. 2848–55.

Kahana B: Umbilical cord prolapse and perinatal outcomes. International Journal of Gynecology and Obstetrics 2004, 84, p. 127–32.

Karbowska J: Trans-fatty acids-effects on coronary heart disease. (Article in Polish) Polski Merkuriusz lekarski, 2011 Jul, 31(181), p. 56–9.

Katz VL, Moos MK, Cefalo RC, Thorp JM Jr, Bowes WA Jr, Wells SD: Group B streptococci. Results of a protocol of antepartum screening and intrapartum treatment. American Journal of Obstetrics and Gynecology, 1994 Feb, 170(2), p. 521–6.

Kayani SI: Uterine rupture after induction of labour in women with previous caesarean section. International Journal of Obstetrics and Gynecology, 2005 Apr, 112, p. 451–5.

Kitzinger S: Birth your Way. DK ADULT, 2002 Jan, p. 238.

Klein MC, Gauthier RJ: Relationship of episiotomy to perineal trauma and morbidity, sexual dysfunction, and pelvic floor relaxation. American Journal of Obstetric and Gynecology, 1994 Sep, 171(3), p. 591–8.

Koebnick C: Long-term ovo-lacto vegetarian diet impairs vitamin B-12 status in pregnant women. Journal of Nutrition, 2004 Dec, 134(12), p. 3319–26.

Koonings PP: Umbilical cord prolapse. A contemporary look. Journal of Reproductive Medicine, 1990, 35, p. 690.

Kühne T: Maternal vegan diet causing a serious infantile neurological disorder due to vitamin B12 deficiency. European Journal of pediatrics, 1991 Jan, 150(3), p. 205–8.

Latva-Pukkila U: Dietary and clinical impacts of nausea and vomiting during pregnancy. Journal of human nutrition and dietetics, 2010 Feb, 23(1), p. 69–77.

Lauener RP et al: Expression of CD14 and Toll-like receptor 2 in farmers' and non-farmers' children. ALEX-Study Group, Lancet, 2002 Aug 10, 360(9331), p. 465–6.

Lin JH: Multi-center study of motherwort injection to prevent postpartum hemorrhage after caesarian section (Article in Chinese). Zhonghua Fu Chan Ke Za Zhi, 2009 Mar, 44(3), p. 175–8.

Lorenz RP et al: Randomised prospective trial comparing ultrasonography and pelvic examination for preterm labor surveillance. American Journal of Obstetrics and Gynecology, 1990 Jun, p. 1603–10.

Louwen F: Vortrag zum Thema Schwangerschaftsdiabetes. Fachtagung „Ernährungsfragen im Säuglingsalter, Darmstadt, 31.10.2012.

Lohmann-Bigelow J: Does Dilation and Curettage Affect Future Pregnancy Outcomes? Ochser Journal, 2007 Winter, 7(4), p. 173–6.

Makrides M: Magnesium supplementation in pregnancy (Review). The Cochrane Collaboration, Wiley, 2012.

Matthews A, Dowswell T, Haas DM et al: Interventions for nausea and vomiting in early pregnancy. Cochrane Database of Systematic Reviews. 2010 Sep, 9, CD007575.

McDonald SJ: Effect of timing of umbilical cord clamping of term infants on maternal and neonatal outcomes. Cochrane Database of Systemic Reviews, 2013 Jul 11, 7:CD004074.

McKenna JJ: Sleeping with Your Baby. A Parent's Guide to Cosleeping. Playtypus Media, LLC, Washington, 2007.

McKenna JJ: Why babies should never sleep alone: A review of the co-sleeping controversy in relation to SIDS, bedsharing and breast feeding. Paediatric Respiratory Reviews, 2005 Jun, 6(2), p. 134–52.

McLean MT: Hemorrhage during pregnancy and childbirth. Midwifery Today, 1998 Dec 1, p. 25–26.

McMath J: Unhindered Living. In: Freeze R: Born free. Unassisted childbirth in North America. Dissertation, University of Iowa, 2008, p. 219, and on McMath's website www.unhinderedliving.com, 2008.

Mellanby E: The Rickets-producing and anti-calcifying action of phytate. Journal of Physiology, 1949 Sep 15, 109(3-4), p. 488–533.

Mercer et al: Labor Outcomes With Increasing Number of Prior Vaginal Births After Cesarean Delivery. Obstetrics and Gynecology, 2008 Feb, 111(2 Pt 1), p. 285–91.

Molloy AM: Maternal vitamin B12 status and risk of neural tube defects in a population with high neural tube defect prevalence and no folic Acid fortification. Pediatrics, 2009 Mar, 123(3), p. 917–23.

Morell SF: The Nourishing Traditions Book of Baby and Childcare. New Trends Publishing Inc, Warsaw, Indiana (USA) 2013.

Mozaffaraian D: Dietary intake of trans fatty acids and systemic inflammation in women. American Journal of Clinical Nutrition, 2004 Apr, 79(4), p. 606–12.

Mozaffaraian D: Trans Fatty Acids and Cardiovascular Disease. New England Journal of Medicine. 2006 Apr, 354, p. 1601–13

Murphy K: Labor and delivery in nulliparous women who present with an unengaged fetal head. Journal of Perinatology, 1998 Mar–Apr, 18(2), p. 122–5.

Nagel R: Cure Tooth Decay. Golden Child Publishing, Ashland, 2011.

Newnham JP et al: Effects of frequent ultrasound during pregnancy: a randomised controlled trial. The Lancet, 1993 Oct, 342(8876), p. 887–91.

Nriagu J: Zinc Deficiency in Human Health. Elsevier, Amsterdam, 2007.

Osman H: Risk factors for the development of striae gravidarum. American Journal of Obstetrics & Gynecology, 2007 Jan, 196(1), 62. p. e1–5.

Ozkan S: Replete vitamin D stores predict reproductive success following in vitro fertilization. Fertility and Sterility, 2010 Sep, 94(4), p. 1314–9.

Phaneuf S et al: Loss of myometrial oxytocin receptors during oxytocin-induced and oxytocin-augmented labour. Journal of Reproduction and Fertility, 2000 Sep, 120(1), p. 91–7.

Phaneuf S. et al: The desensitization of oxytocin receptors in human myometrial cells is accompanied by down-regulation of oxytocin receptor messenger RNA. Journal of Endocrinology, 1997 Jul, 154(1), p. 7–18.

Pötzsch B, Madlener K, Unkrig C, Müller-Berghaus G: Therapie mit Blutkomponenten und Plasmaderivaten in der Geburtshilfe. Gynäkologe 1997, 30(10), S. 782–789.

Price WA: Nutrition and Physical Degeneration. Benediction Classics, Oxford, 2010.

Pschyrembel W: Praktische Geburtshilfe. De Gruyter, Berlin, 1947, S. 46.

Quillin P: Beating Cancer With Nutrition. Nutrition Times Press, Incorporated, Carlsbad, California (USA), 2005.

Ramos JG: Reported calcium intake is reduced in women with preeclampsia. Pregnancy Hypertension, 2006 Oct, 25(3), p. 229–39.

Rath WH: Fruchtwasserembolie – eine interdisziplinäre Herausforderung: Epidemiologie, Diagnostik und Therapie. Deutsches Ärzteblatt, 2014, 111(8), S. 126–32.

Rath WH: Oxytocin und Methylergometrin nach der Geburt – Vorsicht bei der Anwendung!, Frauenarzt, 2008, 49(6), S. 498–503.

Ravnskov U: Is satured fat bad? As published in: De Meester F: Modern Dietary Fat Intakes in Disease Promotion, Nutrition and Health, 2010, Pt 2, p. 109–19.

Reif H, Pomp R: Milchproduktion und Milchvermarktung im Ruhrgebiet 1870–1930. Veröffentlicht im Jahrbuch für Wirtschaftsgeschichte, Berlin, 1996, S. 77–108.

Rockel-Loenhoff A: Rationales Vorgehen bei erschwerter Schulterentwicklung, Österreichische Hebammenzeitung, Apr 2010, S. 12–15.

Rockel-Loenhoff A: Die „Fünf-Minuten-Nahttechnik" eines Dammrisses Grad II. Die Hebamme, März 2012, 25(3), S. 187–190.

Rockenschaub A: Gebären ohne Aberglaube. Facultas, Wien, 2005.

Ronnenberg A: Preconception B-vitamin and homocysteine status, conception, and early pregnancy loss. American Journal of Epidemiology, 2007 Aug, 166(3), p. 304–12.

Ronnenberg A: Preconception Folate and Vitamin B6 Status and Clinical Spontaneous Abortion in Chinese Women. Obstetrics & Gynecology, 2002 Jul, 100(1), p. 107–13.

Saari-Kemppainen A, Karjalainen O, Ylostalo P et al: Ultrasound Screening and perinatal mortality: Controlled trial of systematic one-stage screening in pregnancy. The Helsinki ultrasound trial. Lancet, 1990 Aug, 336(8712), p. 387–91.

Salvesen KÅ: Ultrasound during pregnancy and birthweight, childhood malignancies and neurological development. Ultrasound in Medicine & Biology, 25(7), 1999 Sep, p. 1025–31.

Scheibner V: Evidence of the association between non-specific stress syndrome, DPT injections, and cot death. Immunisation: The Old and the New. Proceedings of the Second National Immunisation Conference, Canbera, Public Health Association of Australia, 1991 May 27–29, p. 90–1.

Schorn MN: Measurement of Blood Loss: Review of the Literature. Journal of midwifery & women's health, 2010 Jan–Feb, 55(1), p. 20–7.

Schrag SJ, Zywicki S: Group B streptococcal disease in the era of intrapartum antibiotic prophylaxis. New England Journal of Medicine, 2000 Jan, 342, p. 15–20.

Schulz-Lobmeyr I et al: Die Kristeller-Technik: Eine prospektive Untersuchung. Geburtshilfe und Frauenheilkunde, 1995, 59, S. 558–61.

Seelig MS: Magnesium deficiency in the pathogenesis of disease. Early Roots of Cardiovascular, Skeletal, and Renal Abnormalities. Plenum Medical Book Company, New York, 1980, Part 2, Chapter 1.

Sherrard EC, Blanco GW: The preparation and analysis of a cattle food consisting of hydrolyzed sawdust. U.S. Department of Agriculture, Forest Service, Forest Products Laboratory, 1920.

Shen J: Association of vitamin B-6 status with inflammation, oxidative stress, and chronic inflammatory conditions: the Boston Puerto Rican Health Study. The American Journal of clinical nutrition, 2010 Feb, 91(2), p. 337–41.

Silver RM: Maternal morbidity associated with multiple repeat cesarean deliveries. Obstetrics and Gynecology, 2006 Jun, 107(6), p. 1226–32.

Smith GC: Use of time to event analysis to estimate the normal duration of human pregnancy. Human Reproduction, Oxford, England, 2001 Jul, 16(7), p. 1497–500.

Spong CY: Risk of uterine rupture and adverse perinatal outcome at term after cesarean delivery. Obstetrics and Gynecology, 2007 Oct, 110(4), p. 801–7.

Stamm J: Winning the Epic Battle Against Stretch Marks. www.stammnutrition.com, 2009 Sep 23. (aufgerufen am 14.5.2014)

Standley CA: Serum Ionized Magnesium Levels in Normal and Preeclamptic Gestation. Obstetrics & Gynecology, 1997 Jan, 89(1), p. 24-7.

Stefansson V: The Fat of the Land. The Macmillian Company, New York, 1960.

Stiftung Weltbevölkerung: Familienplanung rettet Leben. Hannover, 16. Mai 2012.

Supakatisant C: Oral magnesium for relief in pregnancy-induced leg cramps: a randomised controlled trial. Maternal & Child Nutrition, 2012 Aug 22, DOI: 10.1111/j.1740-8709.2012.00440.x.

Sutton J: Understanding and Teaching Optimal Foetal Positioning, Birth Concepts, Tauranga (NZ), 1996.

Tarantal A.F. et al.: Evaluation of the bioeffects of prenatal ultrasound exposure in the Cynomolgus Macaque (Macaca fascicularis). Chapter III in Developmental and Mematologic Studies, Teratology, 1993 Feb, 47(2), p. 159-70.

Tew M: Do obstetric intranatal interventions make birth safer? British Journal of Obstetrics and Gynecology, 1986 Jul, 93(7), p. 659-74.

Torloni MR: Safety of ultrasonography in pregnancy: WHO systematic review of the literature and meta-analysis. Ultrasound in Obstertrics & Gynecology, 2009 May, 33(5), p. 599-608.

Tousoulis D: Endothelial function and inflammation in coronary artery disease. Heart, 2006 Apr, 92(4), p. 441-4.

Troendle J, Zumbrunn M: Knoblauchtherapie bei schwangeren Frauen mit einer vaginalen Streptokokken B Kolonisation – Eine Alternative zur intrapartalen Antibiotikaprophylaxe? Bachelor of Science Hebamme, Berner Fachhochschule Fachbereich Gesundheit, Basel, 6. Aug 2012.

Tully G: www.spinningbabies.com. Maternity House Publishing, Minneapolis, Minnesota (USA), 2012. (abgerufen am 27.3.2014)

Unsworth J, Vause S: Meconium in labour. Obstetrics, Gynecology and Reproductive Medicine, 2010 Oct, 20(10), p. 289-94.

Urbano G: The role of phytic acid in legumes: aninutritient or benefical function? Journal of Physiology and Biochemistry, 2000 Sep, 56(3), p. 283-294.

Watts DL: The Nutritional Relationships of Zinc. Journal of Orthomolecular Medicine, 1988, 3(2), p. 64.

Weiss G et al: Absence of functional Hfe protects mice from invasive Salmonella entericaSerovar Typhimurium infection via induction of lipocalin-2. Vortrag auf der 46th Interscience Conference for Antimicrobial Agents and Chemotherapy (ICAAC), Washington, DC, 2008 Oc 24-27, und dem European Congress for Clinical Microbiology and Infectious Diseases (ECCMID), Helsinki, Finland, 2009 May 16-19.

Weiss PAM: Geburtsrisiko Beckenendlage. In: Feige A, Krause M: Beckenendlage. Urban & Schwarzenberg, München 1998, S. 75-106

Welsch H: Müttersterblichkeit. In: Schneider H, Husslein P, Schneider KM: Die Geburtshilfe. Springer-Verlag, Heidelberg 2011, S. 1207-24.

Weschler T: Taking charge of your fertility, William Morrow Paperbacks, New York City (USA), 2006.

Whiting JWM: Environmental constraints on infant care practices. Handbook of Cross-Cultural Human Development. R. H. Munroe, R. L. Munroe, and B. B. Whiting (eds). Garland STPM Press, New York, 1981, p. 155-79.

White G: Emergency Childbirth. A NAPSAC Publication, Marble Hill, Missouri (USA), 1998, p. 32.

Witlin AG: Magnesium Sulfate Therapy in Preeclampsia and Eclampsia. Obstetrics & Gynecology. 1998 Nov, 92(5), p. 883-9.

Young G: Topical preparations for preventing stretch marks in pregnancy. Cochrane Database of Systematic Review, 2012 Nov 14, 11, CD000066.

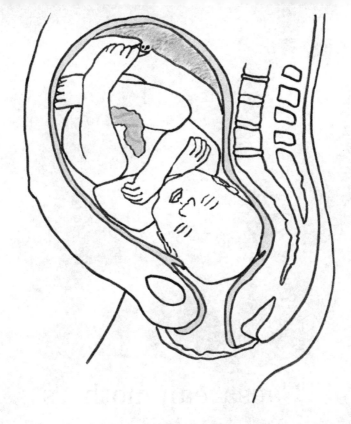

Thanks

This book would not exist without Caroline Oblasser, my publisher. We have never actually met in real life, but have known each other for years in the virtual world, ever since the book project 'Luxus Privatgeburt'. Had she not spurred me on, I'd rather someone else had written this book as life is busy enough with 5 small children and I have been trying to finish my fantasy novel for the last 10 years as well.

But then my love for writing took over. I love writing with all my heart, especially about my favourite subject.

This book would not have been possible without the daily lunchtime nap my kids let me have nearly every day, and my lovely husband who puts up with me sitting in front of the computer or rather working at my back friendly standing desk until the small hours. I very much enjoy those hours of working child-free, without distractions.

And it would definitely not have been possible to write this book had it not been for the births of my children. I have learnt more from those births and the time since than twelve years of schooling and six years at university combined.

I would like to thank Ute Taschner and Anna Rockel-Loenhoff, whose critical expertise helped me to complete this book, as well as my editor Heike Wolter and all the diligent proofreaders. Your additions, comments and corrections have made this book into what it is.

Sincere thanks also to all the families who took the time and effort to share very personal details to be part of this project. Every single one of your stories has moved me and taught me something.

Another special thanks to Deborah Neiger for her translation into the English language. She made it possible for us to take into account UK conventions and particularities in the English edition of this book.

Caroline Oblasser
Photographs by Gudrun Wesp

C-Section Moms

Caesarean mothers in words and photographs

Photo book, guide and a treasure trove of experiences for pregnant women, mothers and obstetricians

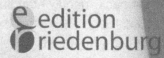

www.editionriedenburg.at

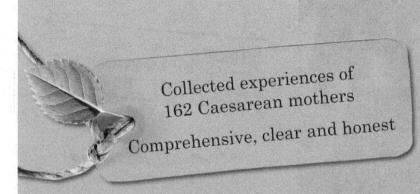

Collected experiences of
162 Caesarean mothers

Comprehensive, clear and honest

Caroline Oblasser (PhD) is the author of several books. Her first daughter was born by Caesarean which was not planned, daughters number 2 and 3 were born at home.

* Mothers with one, two, three or four Caesareans aged between 20 and 77
* Experiences after emergency, elective and planned Caesarean sections
* Spontaneous birth after a C-Section (VBAC)
* Aesthetic photographs of 60 different Caesarean scars
* The "gentle Caesarean section": Photo report of a Caesarean section using the "Misgav Ladach" method
* **PLUS:** Caesarean surgery: Preparation, procedure, aftercare

"A must see and read book for all expectant women, their partners, childbirth educators, doulas, nurses, and all who care for childbearing women!"
(Debra Pascali-Bonaro, "Orgasmic Birth")

"This book should be read by all pregnant women as it speaks the bare truth."
(Marsden Wagner MD, MS)

"We need to tell true stories about caesareans, so that those who come after us aren't caught off guard the way so many of us were."
(Gretchen Humphries, MS DVM; ICAN)

9 783902 943521

ISBN 978-3-902943-52-1

edition riedenburg

editionriedenburg.at

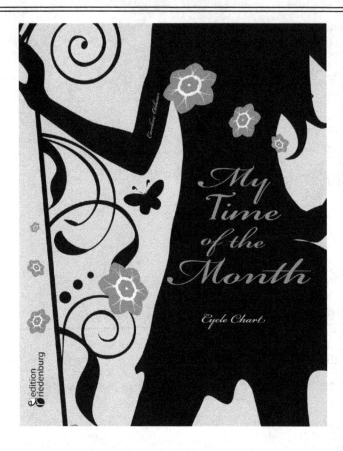

ISBN 978-3-902943-92-7

9 783902 943927

edition **r**iedenburg
editionriedenburg.at

In this cycle diary you will find a chart with 50 templates to record your fertility.

This is what you will record in your charts:

- your waking temperature, location and time of recording as well as type of thermometer
- start of your monthly cycle = first day of your period (also recognisable from the waking temperature)
- duration and intensity of your period
- presence and consistency of your cervical mucus
- estimated time of ovulation
- intercourse
- special events (alcohol consumption, going to bed late, illness/fever, exclusive or complementary breastfeeding, etc)

You can also make note of:

- shortest and longest cycle so far
- personal estimation of fertile days
- general observations regarding menstruation (sanitary protection used, menstrual pain or which pain medications have been used, experiences with freebleeding)
- contraception or trying to conceive
- anything else of importance

The perfect companion for your charting software / mobile app

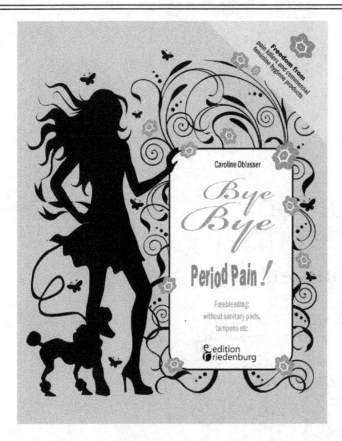

ISBN 978-3-902943-95-8

9 783902 943958

edition riedenburg
editionriedenburg.at

Freedom from pain killers and commercial feminine hygiene products

This is a book for all the girls and women who would like to forego period pain and traditional sanitary protection.

What to expect:

It really does not matter if you have been using tampons, sanitary pads or menstrual cups up to now: you will soon find out how you can leave traditional sanitary protection behind and get rid of your menstrual fluid, in a way convenient to you.

Come on a journey into your innermost body and find out how you can learn to control your cervix and uterus. Once you feel a good connection to both, you will be able to achieve the ideal balance between tension and relaxation – during your menses as well as during times of erotic pleasure.

Contents include:

- How to get started
- Free menstruation and freebleeding: your time of the month without pain
- A small egg birth, every month
- Strengthening erotic sensations and keeping yourself 'shut'
- Cervix, open up!
- The start of your period, trying to conceive and contraception

Plus: 12 months worth of cycle charts to recognise the first day of your period.

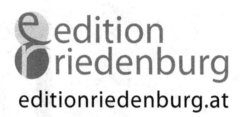

editionriedenburg.at

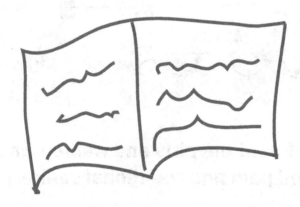

Focussing on
women's health.

CPSIA information can be obtained
at www.ICGtesting.com
Printed in the USA
BVHW090712201222
654548BV00005B/113